Clinical Gastroenterology

Series Editor:
George Y. Wu
University of Connecticut Health Center, Farmington, CT, USA

More information about this series at http://www.springer.com/series/7672

Charan K. Singh

Editor

Gastrointestinal
Interventional Radiology

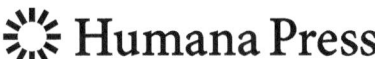 Humana Press

Editor
Charan K. Singh
Department of Interventional Radiology
University of Connecticut Health Center
Farmington, CT
USA

ISSN 2197-7399   ISSN 2197-7704   (electronic)
Clinical Gastroenterology
ISBN 978-3-030-08222-2   ISBN 978-3-319-91316-2   (eBook)
https://doi.org/10.1007/978-3-319-91316-2

This Humana Press imprint is published by the registered company Springer Nature Switzerland AG
The registered company address is: Gewerbestrasse 11, 6330 Cham, Switzerland

Preface

The idea of GI interventional radiology came from my GI colleague trying to educate his fellows how IR could help with the management of variceal bleed. It struck me at the moment that our referring physicians especially at the grassroots level need a refresher on the procedures IR can offer and also update on the new IR techniques, especially since IR has grown rapidly in the last few decades.

The book is authored by experts in their fields and is designed for referring medical, surgical, GI, and IR physicians. The book describes the common day-to-day procedures such as enteral tube feeding and abscess drainage, to more complex interventions like TIPS shunt creation and vessel embolization for GI bleeds, often a lifesaving procedure.

The goal is to briefly describe the indications and basic techniques, help in getting patients prepared for the procedure, and to be aware and manage post-procedure course and any complications.

I acknowledge the authors who took time from their busy schedules to write the chapters. I also thank my parents, my family, daughters, and work colleagues for being an inspiration for academic work. Hopefully, you will enjoy reading the book and it can provide some tips in improving day-to-day patient care.

Farmington, CT, USA   Charan K. Singh

Contents

List of Contributors

Mark Amirault University of New England, Biddeford, Maine, USA

Michael Baldwin, MD University of Connecticut Health Center, Farmington, CT, USA

John A. Cieslak, MD, PhD Northwestern University Feinberg School of Medicine, Chicago, IL, USA

Suvranu Ganguli, MD Department of Interventional Radiology, Massachusetts General Hospital, Boston, MA, USA

Douglas W. Gibson, MD Department of Vascular and Interventional Radiology, University of Connecticut Health Center, Farmington, CT, USA

Harry Griffin, MD University of Connecticut School of Medicine, Farmington, CT, USA

Elizabeth Anne C. Hevert, MD Department of Interventional Radiology, Massachusetts General Hospital, Boston, MA, USA

Samantha Huq, MD Department of Radiology, University of Connecticut School of Medicine, Farmington, CT, USA

Michael E. Langston, MD Department of Radiology, University of Miami - Miller School of Medicine, Jackson Memorial Hospital, Miami, FL, USA

John J. Manov, MD Department of Radiology, University of Miami - Miller School of Medicine, Jackson Memorial Hospital, Miami, FL, USA

Prasoon P. Mohan, MD, MRCS Department of Vascular and Interventional Radiology, University of Miami - Miller School of Medicine, Jackson Memorial Hospital, Miami, FL, USA

Marco Molina, MD University of Connecticut Health Center, Farmington, CT, USA

Charan K. Singh, MD University of Connecticut Health Center, Farmington, CT, USA

Pushpinder Singh Khera, MD, DNB, FRCR Department of Diagnostic and Interventional Radiology, All India Institute of Medical Sciences, Jodhpur, India

Adam Swersky, BS University of Miami Miller School of Medicine, Miami, FL, USA

Elena G. Violari, MD Department of Radiology, University of Connecticut Health Center, Farmington, CT, USA

Chapter 1
Gastrointestinal Imaging

Samantha Huq, Marco Molina, and Charan K. Singh

Abdominal radiograph, ultrasonography (US), computed tomography (CT), and nuclear medicine (NM) scans are often used alone or in combination to provide the maximum diagnostic information and guidance for therapeutic interventions.

Abdominal Radiograph

Abdominal X-ray can be used to detect calcifications. It may be the initial study performed in a patient presenting with right upper quadrant pain. Depending on their composition, gallstones can appear densely calcified, rim calcified, or laminated (Fig. 1.1). Approximately 15–20% of gallstones show up on plain film [1].

Appendicoliths can also be identified using plain films (Fig. 1.2). Layered calcium in the right lower quadrant that moves when comparing supine with upright film is an appendicolith [1].

S. Huq (✉)
Department of Radiology, University of Connecticut School of Medicine, Farmington, CT, USA
e-mail: shuq@uchc.edu

M. Molina
University of Connecticut Health Center, Farmington, CT, USA

C. K. Singh
Department of Interventional Radiology, University of Connecticut Health Center, Farmington, CT, USA

Fig. 1.1 Calcified gallstones identified on plain film. Depending on their composition, gallstones can be densely calcified, laminated in appearance, or rim calcified as in the image shown above

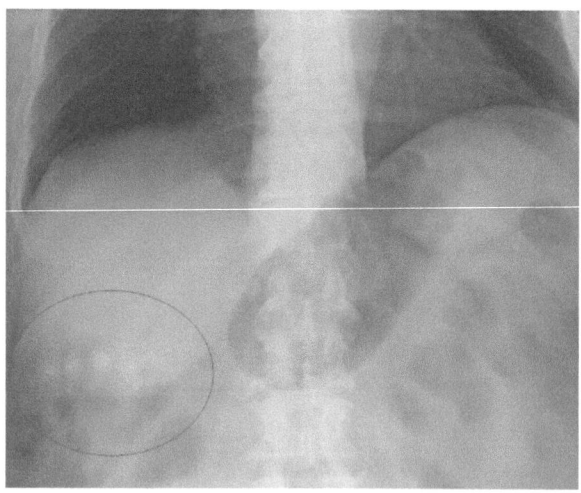

Fig. 1.2 Arrow points to a calcification in the right lower quadrant, which may be an appendicolith or a fecalith. In the setting of right lower quadrant pain, this is suspicious for acute appendicitis

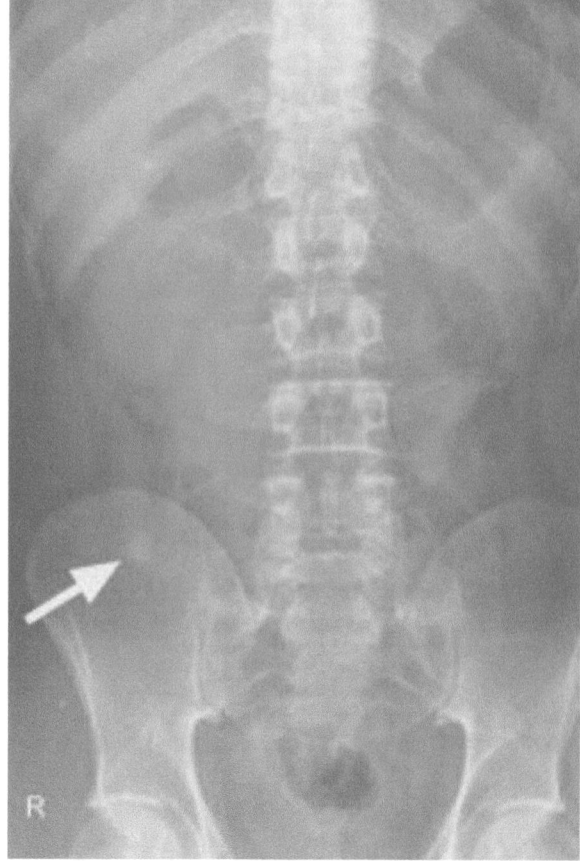

Ultrasonography (US)

US is a valuable diagnostic tool in evaluating patient's with right upper quadrant abdominal pain. It has become the method of choice for identifying cholelithiasis and has been recommended as the study of choice for cholecystitis when an immediate diagnosis is needed (Fig. 1.3). US is nearly 100% accurate in detecting gallbladder calculi. However, the mere presence of cholelithiasis is not diagnostic of acute cholecystitis. The most sensitive US finding in acute cholecystitis is the presence of cholelithiasis in combination with the sonographic Murphy sign, which is defined as maximal abdominal tenderness from pressure of the US probe over the visualized gallbladder. Both gallbladder wall thickening (>3 mm) and pericholecystic fluid are secondary findings. Other less specific findings include gallbladder distension and sludge [2].

Percutaneous gallbladder drainage (cholecystostomy) is indicated for the treatment for acute calculous or acalculous cholecystitis in patients who are not surgical candidates. Cholecystostomy is a temporizing measure for treatment of calculous cholecystitis prior to cholecystectomy whereas it may be a curative measure in acalculous cholecystitis. Under sonographic guidance, percutaneous gallbladder drainage tube is either placed using transhepatic or transperitoneal approach (Figs. 1.4 and 1.5] [2].

Visualization of the biliary tree can be accomplished using US guidance to inject contrast into the biliary system, known as percutaneous transhepatic cholangiography (PTC) (Fig. 1.6). If the biliary system is obstructed, PTC may be used to perform biliary drainage until a more permanent solution to obstruction is performed. PTC is the first step in a number of percutaneous biliary interventions (e.g., percutaneous transhepatic biliary stent placement) [2].

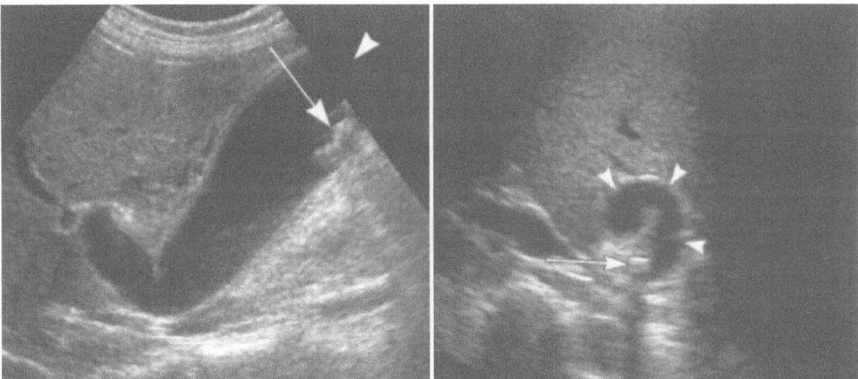

Fig. 1.3 Sagittal sonogram shows stones (arrow) in a distended gallbladder. The patient experienced maximal tenderness when the transducer was pressed over the fundus of the gallbladder (arrowhead) (sonographic Murphy sign) (left). Transverse oblique intercostal sonogram of the neck of the gallbladder (arrowheads) shows an obstructing stone (arrow) (right)

Fig. 1.4 Illustration of percutaneous gallbladder drainage tube

Cholecystostomy (drainage)

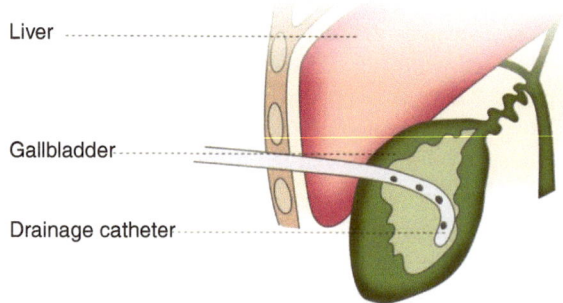

Liver

Gallbladder

Drainage catheter

Fig. 1.5 Longitudinal gray-scale image of the right upper quadrant. US guided needle insertion into the gallbladder lumen. Arrow points to the needle within the gallbladder lumen

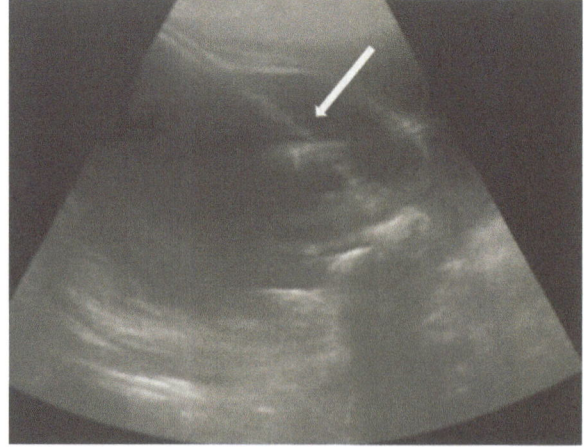

Fig. 1.6 PTC demonstrates the gallbladder (arrow), cystic duct (star), common hepatic duct (solid circle), and the common bile duct (solid arrow)

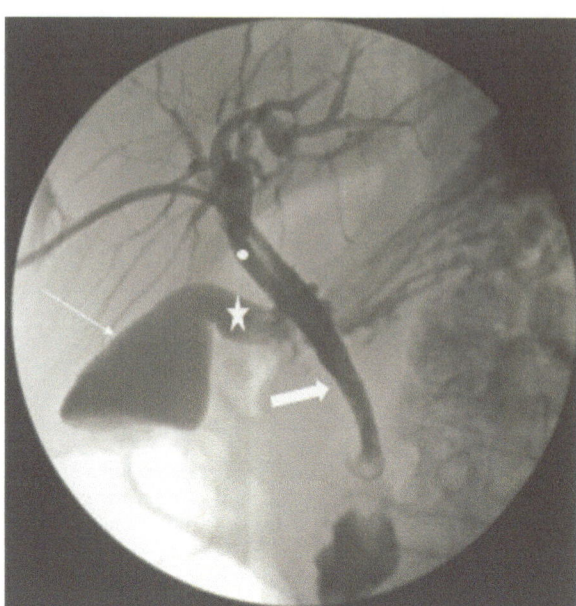

Fig. 1.7 Transverse
transabdominal US
demonstrates a hypoechoic
fluid (arrow) collection
with fluid-fluid level (white
open arrow) representing
an abscess

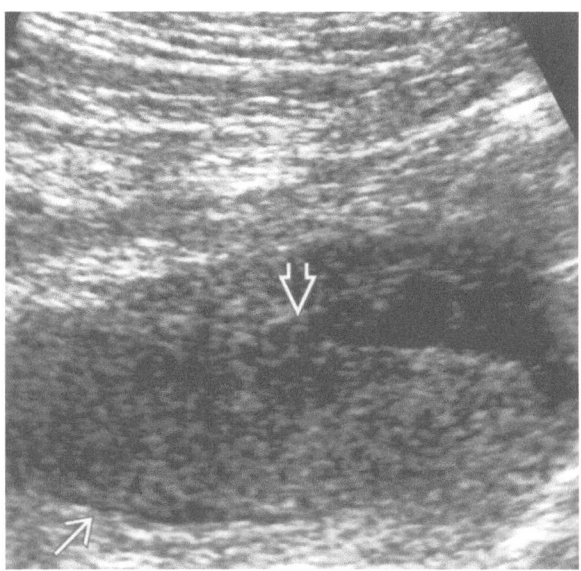

US is also used to evaluate palpable abdominal masses or fluid collections such as an abscess (Fig. 1.7). It can be used to perform biopsies and abscess drainage. US provides the advantage of continuous visualization of the needle course toward the target. The speed, portability, cost-effectiveness, and lack of ionizing radiation make US a preferred technique. The disadvantages are that images may be hindered by technical factors such as patient obesity or the presence of bowel gas [3].

Computed Tomography (CT)

Gastrointestinal (GI) bleeding can be classified as upper GI (bleeding source proximal to the ligament of Treitz) and lower GI (bleeding source distal to the ligament of Treitz). Endoscopy is the best initial procedure for acute upper GI bleeding, as it can be both diagnostic and therapeutic. For lower GI bleeding, a hemodynamically stable patient should first be evaluated by mesenteric CT angiogram (CTA) or nuclear medicine tagged red blood cell scan to localize the bleed as they are both more sensitive then angiography. CTA provides a relatively noninvasive and effective way of localizing the source of bleeding (Fig. 1.8) [4].

However, a hemodynamically unstable patient with clinical evidence of current GI bleeding should directly go to angiography. Angiography can provide the opportunity for therapeutic intervention at the time of diagnosis.

CT is also the choice for evaluating patients who present with fever and suspected abscess. CT is best suited for small and deep lesions especially those involving the retroperitoneum. Using CT, both the depth of the lesion and the path angle can be determined prior to performing biopsy or abscess drainage (Fig. 1.9). CT allows for the unequivocal visualization of the needle tip and surrounding structures thereby avoiding nearby structures [4].

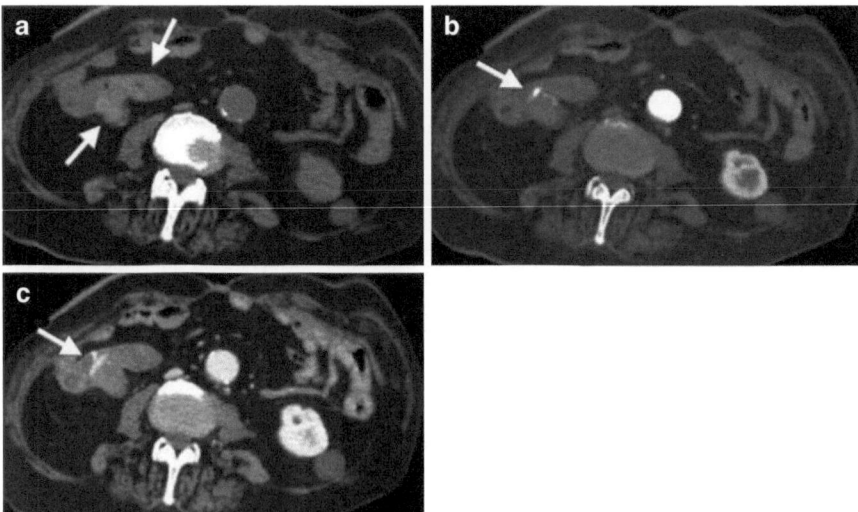

Fig. 1.8 (a) Axial unenhanced CTA image shows intraluminal hyperattenuation (arrows). (b, c) Axial arterial phase (b) and portal venous phase (c) CTA images show an intraluminal jet (arrow) of contrast material in the arterial phase, which changes in size and morphology in the portal venous phase. This represents an active GI bleed

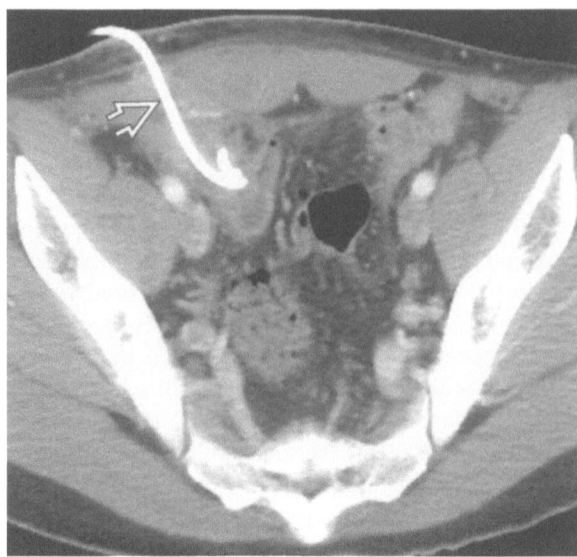

Fig. 1.9 Axial contrast-enhanced CT demonstrates pigtail catheter (white open arrow) placed percutaneously in encapsulated fluid collection in the right lower quadrant from a ruptured appendix

Radionuclide Scanning

When the diagnosis of acute cholecystitis is equivocal on US, hepatobiliary scan can be performed, which has nearly 100% accuracy in identifying acute cholecystitis. Technetium 99m hepatobiliary iminodiacetic acid (HIDA) is taken up in the liver and excreted in the bile. Visualization of the liver, the gallbladder, and the biliary tree is thereby accomplished (Fig. 1.10). If visualization of the gallbladder within an hour of administration of the radionuclide is accomplished, a diagnosis of acute cholecystitis is virtually excluded, even in acalculous disease. Hepatobiliary scanning has been demonstrated to be 95–100% specific and sensitive in diagnosing acute cholecystitis, respectively [5].

In addition to CTA, lower GI bleeds can also be detected using erythrocytes labelled with technetium-99m after which serial scintigraphy is performed (tagged red blood cell scan) to detect focal collections of radiolabeled material (Fig. 1.11). It can help localize the general area of active bleeding to guide subsequent treatment course including angiography or surgery [6].

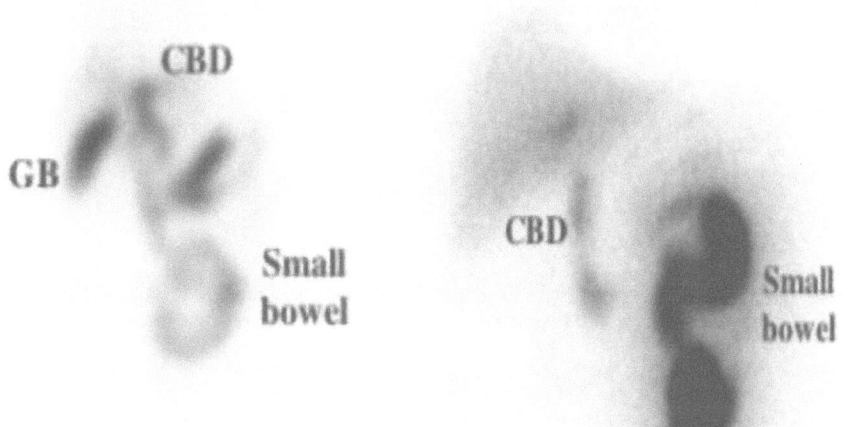

Fig. 1.10 Normal HIDA scan (left) shows tracer in the gallbladder (GB), common bile duct (CBD), and the small bowel. On the right, no filling of the GB, tracer is present in the CBD and the small bowel indicating acute cholecystitis

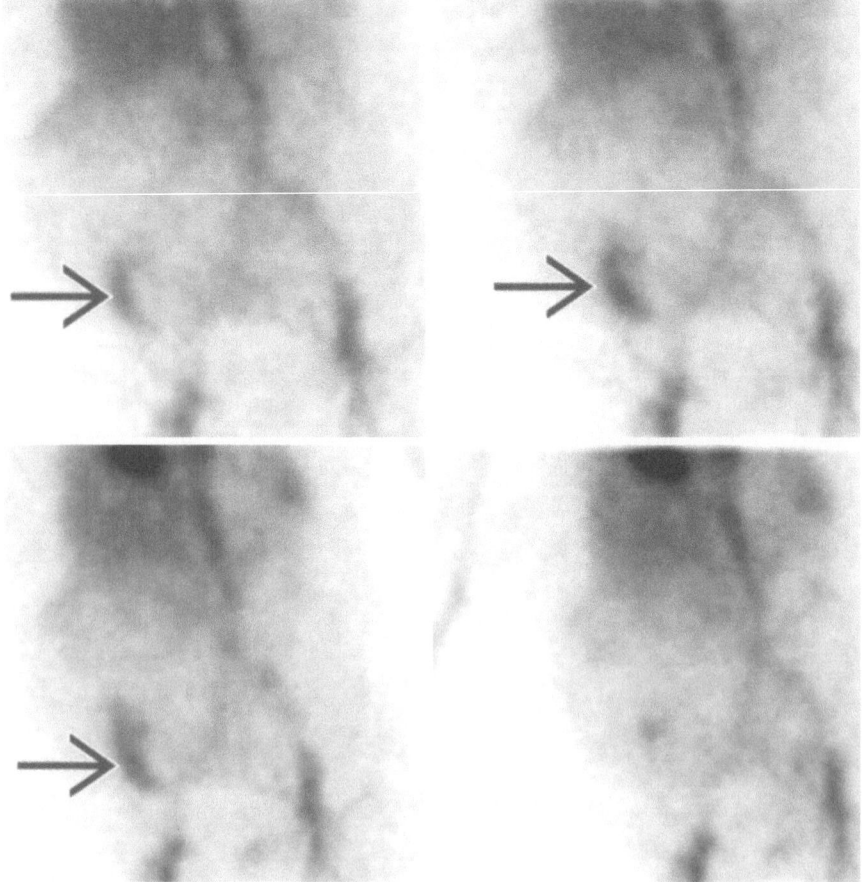

Fig. 1.11 Technetium 99m tagged RBC scan (selected sequential images) shows accumulation of radiotracer within the cecum and ascending colon (arrows) indicating active bleeding

References

1. Wiest P, Roth P. Fundamentals of emergency radiology. Philadelphia: W.B. Saunders Company; 1996.
2. Hanbidge A, Buckler P, O'Malley M, Wilson S. Imaging evaluation for acute pain in the right upper quadrant. Radiographics. 2004;24(4):1117–35.
3. Rosen P, et al. Diagnostic radiology in emergency medicine. St. Louis: Mosby-Year Book, Inc.; 1992.
4. Artigas J, Milagros M, Soto F, Esteban H, Pinilla I, Guillen E. Multidetector CT angiography for acute gastrointestinal bleeding: technique and findings. Radiographics. 2013;33:1453–70.
5. Wood B, Wood S. Radiology. Baltimore: Williams & Wilkins; 1998.
6. Juhl J, et al. Essentials of radiologic imaging. Philadelphia: Lippincott-Raven Publishers; 1998.

Chapter 2
Enteric Feeding and Decompression Tubes

John A. Cieslak, Elena G. Violari, and Douglas W. Gibson

Nasogastric/Nasoenteric Tube Placement

Gastric intubation via the nasal passage (i.e., nasogastric) is a common procedure that provides access to the stomach for various indications. The majority of nasogastric/nasoenteric tubes are inserted on the ward level. In difficult cases, insertion under fluoroscopic guidance is undertaken. A silicone catheter known as a nasogastric (NG) tube is used for the procedure. Diagnostic indications for NG placement include evaluation for upper GI bleeding, aspiration for evaluation of gastric contents, and administration of contrast to the gastrointestinal tract. Therapeutic indications for NG placement include gastric decompression after endotracheal intubation or in the setting of small-bowel obstruction, aspiration of gastric contents after toxic ingestion, feeding, administration of medication, and bowel irrigation. Contraindications for NG placement include mid-face trauma and recent nasal surgery (absolute contraindications) and coagulation abnormalities, esophageal varices, esophageal stricture, and recent alkaline ingestion (relative contraindications).

J. A. Cieslak (✉)
Northwestern University Feinberg School of Medicine, Chicago, IL, USA
e-mail: john.cieslak@northwestern.edu

E. G. Violari
Department of Radiology, University of Connecticut Health Center, Farmington, CT, USA
e-mail: violari@uchc.edu

D. W. Gibson
Department of Vascular and Interventional Radiology, University of Connecticut Health Center, Farmington, CT, USA
e-mail: dgibson@uchc.edu

© Springer International Publishing Switzerland 2018
C. K. Singh (ed.), *Gastrointestinal Interventional Radiology*, Clinical Gastroenterology, https://doi.org/10.1007/978-3-319-91316-2_2

As infusion of feeding solutions beyond the pylorus presumably lessens the chance of aspiration, placement of enteral tubes into the duodenum or preferably into the jejunum is a major goal [1]. A variety of nasoenteral tubes are available (see below), and techniques for their placement include blind approaches that use periodic abdominal films to verify placement or fluoroscopic and endoscopic methods [1–12]. Blind placement of feeding tubes with weighted tips followed by plain films of the abdomen to document their position is often done initially. However, this method is less effective than fluoroscopic or endoscopically guided techniques and is more time consuming [2, 3].

Choosing the Correct Enteric Tube

The correct choice of enteric tube depends greatly on the indication for the tube. If the patient has a small-bowel obstruction and decompression is required, then a Salem Sump catheter would be the best choice. If the patient had a recent toxic ingestion and gastric lavage is required, the Salem Sump would also be the best choice. If the patient requires long-term enteric feeding and is at risk for aspiration, then post-pyloric placement of a Dobhoff tube would be a good choice. Short-term enteral nutrition in a patient with low risk for aspiration can be accomplished with the non-weighted Kangaroo tube in a nasogastric position. Types of enteric tubes and their uses are listed below and summarized in Table 2.1:

• *Levin catheter*, which is a single-lumen, small-bore enteric tube. It can be placed in a nasogastric or nasoduodenal position. It is more appropriate for administration of medication or nutrition than decompression, though the manufacturer states that it can also be used for gastrointestinal aspiration.

Table 2.1 Comparison of common enteral tubes

	Levin catheter	Salem Sump	Dobhoff tube	Kangaroo tube
Most common indication	Administration of medication of nutrition	Gastric decompression	Enteral feeding (long-term, risk of aspiration)	Enteral feeding (short-term, minimal risk of aspiration)
Caliber	Small-bore	Large-bore	Small-bore	Small-bore
Positioning	Nasogastric or nasoduodenal	Nasogastric	Post-pyloric (nasoduodenal)	Nasogastric
Photo				

- *Salem Sump catheter*—a large-bore NG tube with double lumen—the most common nasogastric tube. This design avails for aspiration in one lumen and venting in the other to reduce negative pressure and prevents gastric mucosa from being drawn into the catheter (Fig. 2.1). The design and large size of this catheter make it ideal for suction and decompression.
- *Dobhoff tube*—a small-bore NG tube inserted using a stylet and with a weight at the end intended to pull it distally into the bowel by gravity and peristalsis during insertion, most often used for post-pyloric positioning and administration of enteral nutrition. It can be left in place for 6 weeks or more (Fig. 2.2). The catheter is small in caliber and is not suitable to be used for suction.
- *Kangaroo tube*—a small-bore, non-weighted catheter intended for short-term administration of nasogastric enteral nutrition (Fig. 2.3). It can be left in place for 3 days.

Fig. 2.1 Salem Sump nasogastric tube

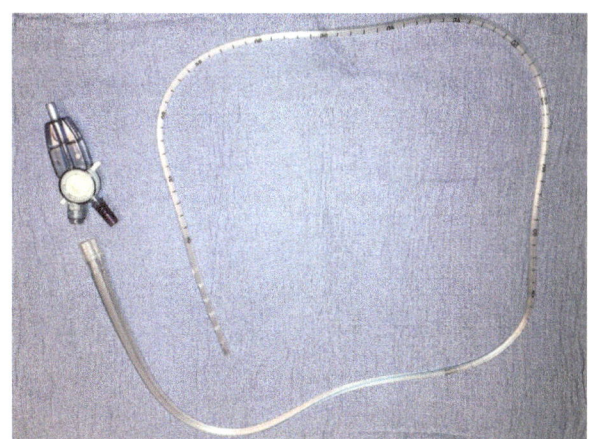

Fig. 2.2 Dobhoff style enteric feeding tube, weighted

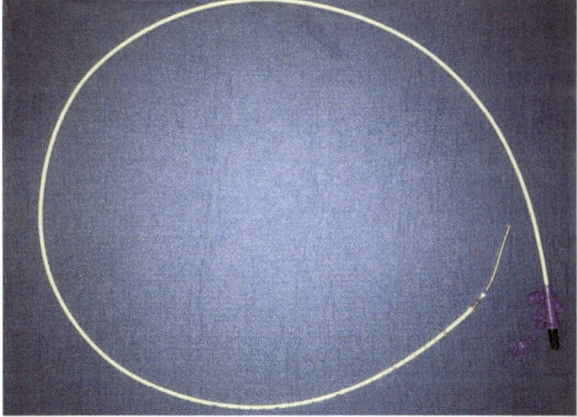

Fig. 2.3 Kangaroo tube, non-weighted

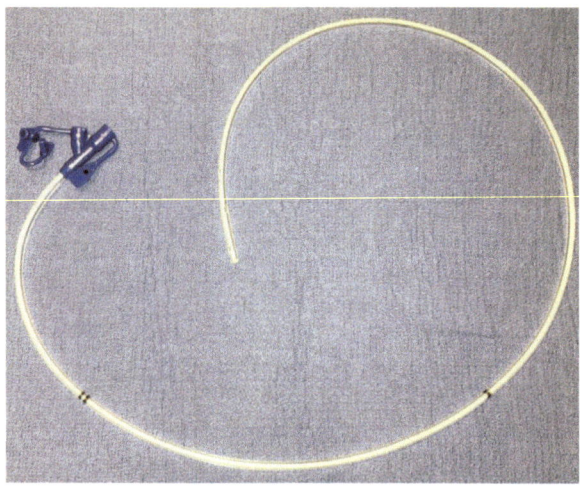

Pre-procedure

Not much pre-procedural preparation is required before the placement of a nasoenteric tube. Typically the patient is already NPO given the indications for tube placement. The patient should be asked if they have allergy to topical anesthetic (lidocaine, xylocaine, etc.). If the procedure is done with the assistance of fluoroscopic guidance, consent may need to be obtained depending on institutional guidelines.

Procedural Details

Before an NG tube is inserted, it must be measured from the tip of the patient's nose and looped around the ear and then down to roughly 5 cm below the xiphoid process. The tube is then marked at this level to ensure that the tube has been inserted far enough into the patient's stomach. Before insertion, inspect each naris for patency, noting any polyps, irritated mucosa, deviation of the nasal septum, or other problems that may complicate insertion [13]. Instill viscous xylocaine 2% jelly (for oral use) down the more patent nostril with the head tilted backward (assuming there is no history of allergy to xylocaine), ask the patient to sniff and swallow to anesthetize the nasal and oropharyngeal mucosa, and then wait 5–10 min for the xylocaine to take effect. The first 2–4 in. of the tube should also be lubricated with the xylocaine jelly.

The tube should be then be inserted while being directed straight posteriorly as it moves through the nasal cavity and down into the throat. When the tube enters the oropharynx, the patient may gag and should be instructed to swallow water through a straw or perform dry swallows. If resistance is met, rotate tube slowly with downward advancement but do not force the tube. If there is a change in the patient's respiratory status, withdraw the tube immediately. If there is minimal resistance, the tube can then be advanced into the expected location within the stomach, however,

Fig. 2.4 Fluoroscopic placement of a weighted Dobhoff tube into the correct position within the third segment of the duodenum

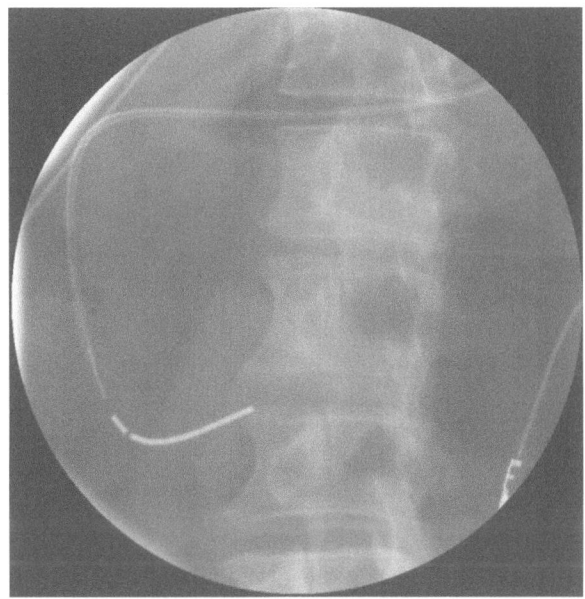

great care must be taken to ensure that the tube has not passed through the larynx into the trachea and down into the bronchi. One method to ensure gastric positioning is to aspirate some fluid and test it with pH paper. If the pH is 4 or below, then the tube is in correct position, but even these should always be confirmed with abdominal radiographs. If the tube is intended for suction, connect the free end of the tubing to suction and set the type of suction and pressure as prescribed [2–4]. If persistent difficulty try using a 5 Fr Kumpe catheter with a glidewire with lateral view of the pharynx to guide the wire posteriorly into oropharynx.

If placing a Dobhoff tube, then the feeding tube has a weighted metal tip and a guidewire to assist in insertion. The tip of Dobhoff tubes should be placed into a post-pyloric position into the second or third portion of the duodenum (Fig. 2.4) [1, 4, 14]. Most tubes, however, are placed into the stomach (Fig. 2.5). If performed without fluoroscopic guidance, a post-insertion radiograph centered on the lower chest/upper abdomen should be performed to confirm positioning. When using fluoroscopic guidance, confirmation of tube positioning is achieved in real time as the tube is directed into a post-pyloric position [4, 6]. If questions of tube migration or position change arise later, repeat radiographs can be performed.

There is an approximately 2% risk of tracheopulmonary complication from insertion of a nasoenteric tube, including inadvertent insertion into the tracheobronchial tree—if this happens, the tube is more likely to enter the right main stem bronchus and right lower lobe bronchus because of the wider diameter and straighter course of the bronchus compared to the left [7]. Additionally, there is a small risk of perforation of the pleura by the guidewire or tube resulting in pneumothorax. There is a risk of aspiration with tubes positioned too proximally. For example, a Dobhoff tube positioned in a pre-pyloric position within the stomach would present a risk for aspiration (Fig. 2.5). Finally, there is a very small but demonstrable risk of intracranial tube placement [4, 6, 8].

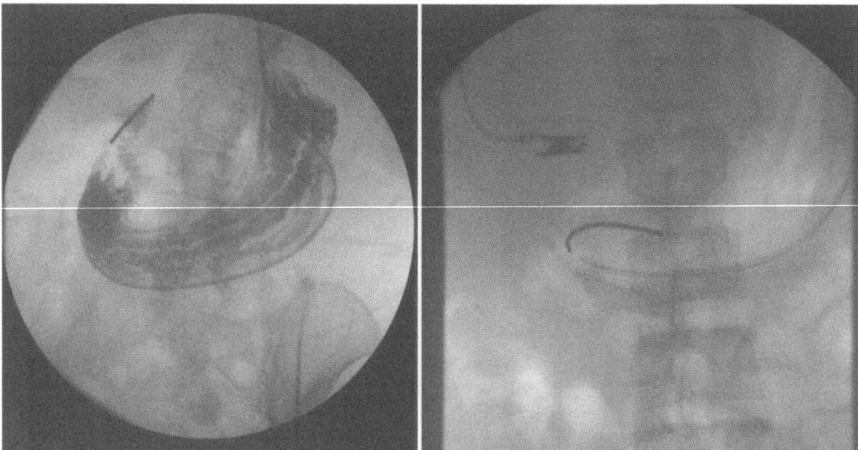

Fig. 2.5 Malpositioned prepyloric Dobhoff feeding tubes within the gastric antrum directed superiorly (left) and within the gastric antrum curled back on itself (right)

Post-procedure

Post-procedurally, the most important steps to take are to secure the enteric tube to the patient and to confirm its position. If the enteric tube is inserted by radiology using fluoroscopic guidance, then the position of its tip will be known in real time within the fluoroscopy suite. If a nasogastric tube is inserted on the floor, its position within the stomach can be confirmed by the return of gastric contents with pH equal to or <4. If there is any resistance to aspiration or flushing of the tube, or any question as to the position of the nasogastric tube, then a portable abdominal radiograph should be obtained to verify that the tip and proximal side hole are distal to the gastroesophageal junction and that the tube is not coiled upon itself within the stomach or distal esophagus. Furthermore, the position of any post-pyloric tube placed without fluoroscopic assistance should always be confirmed with abdominal radiographs. Once the tube is in place, it can then be hooked to low-intermittent suction (for gastric decompression) or to the appropriate enteral nutrition to administer the correct amount of calories and volume per hour as usually determined from consulting the inpatient nutritionist. To prevent clot, the enteral tube should be flushed with 30 cc warm water daily after administration of medications or nutrition. If the enteral tube becomes clogged or will not withdraw easily, it can be flushed forcibly with 30–60 cc warm water using a syringe and a Christmas tree adaptor. These solutions should be allowed to sit 5 min before repeated flushing attempts are made. Additionally, enzymatic de-clogging treatments are available, such as Clog Zapper or Viokace which are mixed with a solution of sodium bicarbonate and administered using a syringe [15].

Example Procedural Note

Nasogastric Tube Placement
Clinical information:

Comparison: (None)

Findings: Viscous lidocaine 2% gel was applied to the (right/left) nares. A [___] French nasogastric tube was advanced under fluoroscopic guidance into the stomach. The proximal side hole was seen below the level of the gastroesophageal junction. Placement was further confirmed with administration of a small amount of water soluble contrast through the tube. The NG tube was flushed with water and secured using adhesive tape. The patient tolerated the procedure well with no immediate complications.

Fluoroscopy time: [___] minutes

Impression: Nasogastric tube in appropriate position and ready for immediate use

References

1. Grant JP, Curtas MS, Kelvin FM. Fluoroscopic placement of nasojejunal feeding tubes with immediate feeding using a nonelemental diet. JPEN J Parenter Enter Nutr. 1983;7:299–303.
2. Ramos SM, Lindine P. Inexpensive, safe and simple nasoenteral intubation: an alternative for the cost conscious. JPEN J Parenter Enteral Nutr. 1986;10:78–81.
3. Thurlow PM. Bedside enteral feeding tube placement into duodenum and jejunum. JPEN J Parenter Enter Nutr. 1986;10:104–5.
4. Frederick PR, Miller MH, Morrison WJ. Feeding tube for fluoroscopic placement. Radiology. 1982;145:847.
5. Silk DBA, Aees AG, Keohane PP, Attrill H. Clinical efficacy and design changes of "fine bore" nasogastnc feeding tubes: a seven-year experience involving 809 intubations in 403 patients. JPEN J Parenter Enter Nutr. 1987;1(1):378–83.
6. Prager A, Laboy V, venus B, Mathru M. Value of fluoroscopic during transpyloric intubation. Crit Care Med. 1986;1(4):151–2.
7. Woodall BH, Winfield DF, Bisset GS 3rd. Inadvertent tracheobronchial placement of feeding tubes. Radiology. 1987;165:727–9.
8. Gutierrez ED, Balfe DM. Fluoroscopically guided nasoenteric feeding tube placement: results of a 1-year study. Radiology. 1991;178:759–62.
9. Lewis BS, Mauer K, Bush A. The rapid placement of jejunal feeding tubes: the Seldinger technique applied to the gut. Gastrointest Endosc. 1990;36:139–41.
10. Chung ASK, Denbesten L. Improved technique for placement of intestinal feeding tube with the fiberoptic endoscope. Gut. 1976;17:264–6.
11. Pleatman MA, Naunheim KS. Endoscopic placement of feeding tubes in assisted the critically ill patient. Surg Gynecol Obstet. 1987;165:69–70.
12. Aives DA, LeRoy JL, Hawkins ML, Bowden TA Jr. Endoscopically nasojejunal feeding tube placement. Am Surg. 1989;55:88–91.
13. Durai R, Ramya V, Philip C. Nasogastric tubes 1: insertion technique and confirming position. Nurs Times. 2009;105:16.

14. Barclay AR, Beattie LM, Weaver LT, Wilson DC. Systematic review: medical and nutritional interventions for the management of intestinal failure and its resultant complications in children. Aliment Pharmacol Ther. 2011;33:175–84.
15. Fisher C, Blalock B. Clogged feeding tubes: a clinician's thorn. Pract Gastroenterol. 2014;127:16–22.

Chapter 3
Gastrostomy and Gastrojejunostomy

Prasoon P. Mohan, John J. Manov, Michael E. Langston, and Charan K. Singh

Introduction

Percutaneous radiological gastrostomy (PRG) is a common procedure that allows for enteral feeding in patients for whom oral intake is impossible or inadequate. PRG can also be used for decompression of the gastrointestinal tract in case of obstruction due to various reasons [1]. Compared to surgical gastrostomy, PRG is a minimally invasive procedure with greatly reduced procedural morbidity and cost while ensuring a high rate of technical success. Surgical gastrostomy was first performed in 1837, becoming a routine method by the end of the nineteenth century. The requirements for general anesthesia and a high surgical morbidity led to the development in 1980 of percutaneous endoscopic gastrostomy (PEG). In 1983, percutaneous radiological gastrostomy was first performed using fluoroscopy, allowing for a minimal amount of anesthesia and invasiveness. Together, PEG and PRG techniques have all but replaced surgical gastrostomy for the vast majority of patients [2].

P. P. Mohan (✉)
Department of Vascular and Interventional Radiology, University of Miami - Miller School of Medicine, Jackson Memorial Hospital, Miami, FL, USA
e-mail: PXP136@med.miami.edu

J. J. Manov · M. E. Langston
Department of Radiology, University of Miami - Miller School of Medicine, Jackson Memorial Hospital, Miami, FL, USA
e-mail: jjm86@med.miami.edu; mel59@med.miami.edu

C. K. Singh
Department of Interventional Radiology, University of Connecticut Health Center, Farmington, CT, USA

© Springer International Publishing Switzerland 2018
C. K. Singh (ed.), *Gastrointestinal Interventional Radiology*, Clinical Gastroenterology, https://doi.org/10.1007/978-3-319-91316-2_3

Terminology

The term percutaneous gastrostomy refers to techniques in which the catheter is placed in the stomach for feeding purposes. Gastrojejunostomy or transgastric jejunostomy refers to the placement of a catheter via a gastric access through the pylorus and duodenum into the jejunum where the tip is placed. Rarely, direct percutaneous access to the jejunum is obtained without a gastric stoma (direct jejunostomy) [3].

There are two common types of percutaneous gastrostomy placed under radiological guidance. The "pull-type" gastrostomy tubes are large bore (20–24 Fr) and have a mushroom retention device that provides the most secure retention. Their placement involves passage of a wire from the stomach under radiologic guidance into the esophagus and mouth, and the tube is pulled into the stomach using the wire [4] (Fig. 3.1). This method poses a potential risk for stomal infection or tumor seeding due to passage of tube through the oral cavity. The second "push-gastrostomy" is small-bore (12–16 Fr) tubes inserted directly through the abdominal wall into the stomach. These have a pigtail or internal balloon as retention, are less secure, and often require gastropexy during tube placement (Figs. 3.2 and 3.3).

Gastrojejunostomy tubes are placed in certain circumstances. If direct jejunal feeding is required due to risk of aspiration, a single small-bore transgastric jejunal tube is placed (Fig. 3.4). In cases of gastric outlet obstruction where simultaneous gastric decompression is required, a double bore gastrojejunostomy tube with separate openings in stomach and jejunum are placed. The stomach port is used for decompression and jejunal port for feeding (Fig. 3.5).

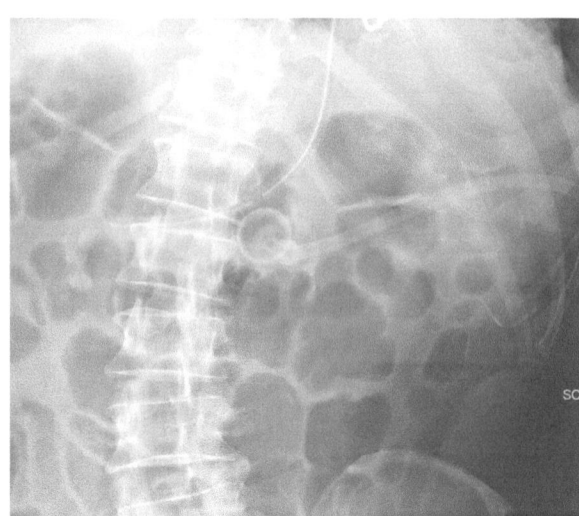

Fig. 3.1 Bumper retention (mushroom), large-bore (20–24 Fr) gastrostomy tube. These are placed using peroral technique with image or endoscopic guidance

It is important to know differences between gastrostomy and gastrojejunostomy feedings. The GJ tube feeds are continuous low-volume feeds that require a specialized pump with a significant burden on the patient and family members. Gastric feedings can be given in boluses and easier to prepare and administer. Medications should be given via the G-tube port into the stomach because the bio-availability is known for gastric delivery and not jejunal delivery.

Fig. 3.2 Pigtail gastrostomy tube (12–16 Fr Wills-Oglesby)

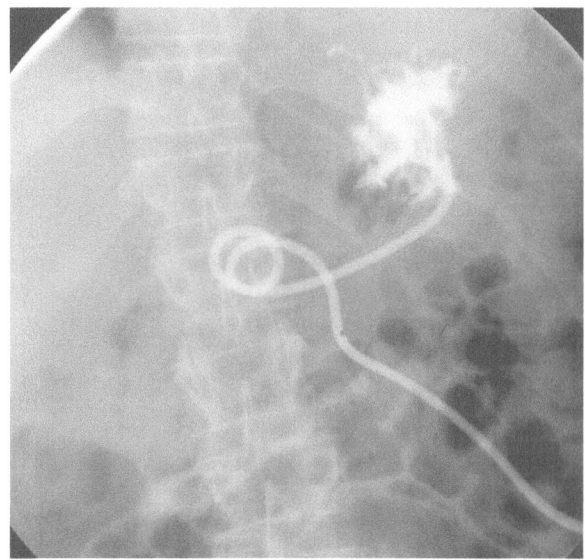

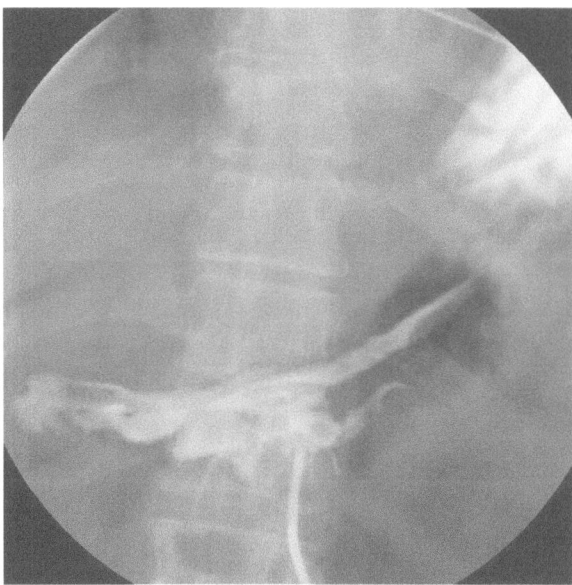

Fig. 3.3 Balloon retention MIC gastrostomy tube, variable size. Good as replacement tubes since easier to place via existing track

Fig. 3.4 Transgastric single-bore jejunostomy tube for jejunal feeds (Shetty/Carey-Coons type)

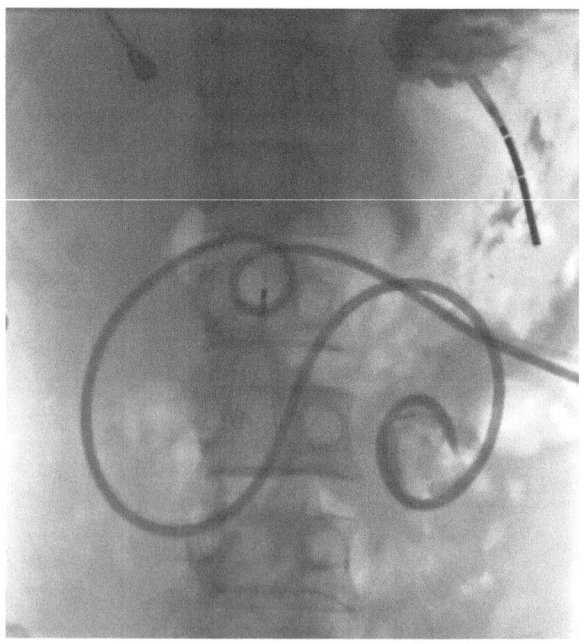

Fig. 3.5 MIC type gastrojejunostomy tube with separate gastric and jejunal ports. Incidental jejunal stent

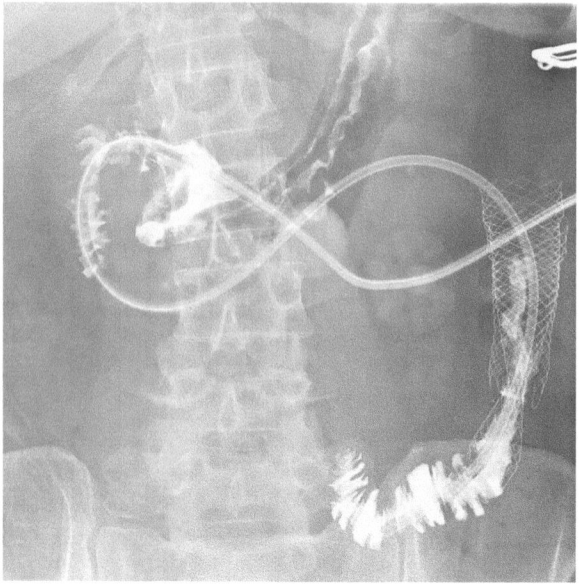

Indications

The most common indication for gastrostomy placement is a requirement for long-term enteral feeding (Table 3.1). Enteral feeding has a much lower incidence of complications compared to total parenteral nutrition. Gastrostomy tubes are also used in patients who require long-term decompression of the stomach or intestines. Gastrostomy tubes allow the avoidance of the complications of long-term nasogastric tube placement, which can include nasal alar ulceration, rhinosinusitis, esophageal stricture, and gastroesophageal reflux, which may result in aspiration pneumonia [2].

Abnormal swallowing mechanism is the most common pathology necessitating long-term enteral feeding. This includes patients with deficits in swallowing function secondary to cerebrovascular accident or traumatic brain injury. Gastrostomy is well tolerated in patients with dysphagic stroke [5]. Current stroke management guidelines recommend a trial of nasogastric feeding for a period of up to 3 weeks before placement of a gastrostomy tube [6]. Patients with malignancies of the head and neck or esophagus may require gastrostomies permanently or temporarily after surgical resection [7]. Percutaneous radiologic gastrostomy has been found to have a lower complication rate and lower procedure-related mortality rate in this population [8]. Percutaneous endoscopic gastrostomy is not widely used in esophageal cancer patients due to reduced technical feasibility due to esophageal obstruction and the potential for spread of tumor cells to the stoma site. Percutaneous radiologic gastrostomy has been found to be feasible, safe, and useful in this population [9].

Table 3.1 Indications for gastrostomy/gastrojejunostomy

Indications for gastrostomy/gastrojejunostomy
Abnormal swallowing mechanism
Cerebrovascular accident
Traumatic brain injury
Amyotrophic lateral sclerosis
Oral/esophageal obstruction
Esophageal cancer
Head and neck malignancy
Post aerodigestive tract surgery
Bowel decompression
Chronic malignant small bowel obstruction
Unrelieved gastric outlet obstruction
Miscellaneous
Inflammatory bowel disease
Radiation enteritis
Scleroderma
Short gut syndrome

Gastrostomy tubes are also frequently used in the palliation of primary neurological disease, with the aim of increasing nutritional support while reducing aspiration. Gastrostomy placement is now considered the standard of care for patients with amyotrophic lateral sclerosis who require alternatives to oral intake. Migration of the stomach into the thorax due to diaphragmatic laxity in this condition can make PEG placement difficult or impossible. PRG has been found in one study to have a significantly higher success rate and better safety profile than PEG for this patient population [10]. PRG has been used to facilitate enteral administration of carbidopa/levodopa effectively in patients with advanced Parkinson's disease [11]. The placement of gastrostomy tubes in patients with dementia is controversial. It is generally not recommended in more advanced cases because of a lack of benefit and high risk of complications [12]. It has been found that gastrostomy feeding does not reduce the incidence of aspiration pneumonia in patients with dementia [13]. It is thought by many that the risk of aspiration pneumonia is reduced with gastrojejunostomy feeding, and it has been reported that modification of percutaneous gastrostomies to gastrojejunostomies reduced the rate of aspiration pneumonia in patients with dysphagia secondary to dementia [14].

Less common indications for enteral feeding through a gastrostomy include diseases in which intestinal function is compromised such as inflammatory bowel disease, radiation enteritis, scleroderma, or the short gut syndrome [7]. Gastrostomy has been safe and effective for nutritional support in Crohn's disease, in spite of misconceptions among some clinicians that inflammatory bowel disease is a strict contraindication to gastrostomy placement [15]. Gastrostomies are also performed for children with severe lung disease (e.g., cystic fibrosis) or cardiac disease in which patients lose the exercise capacity required for alimentation [16].

At most centers, the decision of gastrostomy placement technique will depend primarily on operator experience and availability. Endoscopic placement is more likely to fail in obese patients, patients with a high stomach, and patients with esophageal or oropharyngeal pathology. Endoscopic placement may be impossible in patients with a high grade of esophageal obstruction and is contraindicated in the setting of potentially curable aerodigestive malignancies for the fear of tract seeding of tumor cells [17].

Apart from enteral nutrition, bowel decompression in case of unrelieved obstruction is also an indication for PRG. This requires the use of large bore tubes for optimal relief of nausea and cramping. Percutaneous radiologic gastrostomy is often preferred to other modalities in these patients due to its lower invasiveness in these patients, who usually have a malignancy and are quite ill [2]. Improved medical management of malignant bowel obstruction has made palliative decompression gastrostomy a less common procedure [18]. When necessary and successful, gastrostomy can allow for the care of terminally ill patients at home or in hospice as opposed to an acute care setting. The presence of peritoneal disease and ascites can make gastrostomy placement technically challenging in patients with gastrointestinal malignancies. One study of 89 oncology patients found an initial technical success rate of 72% for the placement of venting gastrostomies under fluoroscopic guidance [19].

Gastrostomy is usually sufficient for both feeding and decompressive purposes. Primary gastrojejunostomy is recommended in those cases in which there is a high degree of concern for possible aspiration of enteral feeds. Patients with a history of neurological disease, previous aspiration, gastroesophageal reflux, or known hiatal hernia may be considered at high risk for aspiration. Patients who have evidence of reflux of feed or possible aspiration after primary gastrostomy should be considered candidates for conversion to gastrojejunostomy. The use of a dual-lumen tube with a gastric opening to suction and a jejunal opening for feedings may be indicated in the setting of gastric outlet obstruction [18]. Primary percutaneous jejunostomy is indicated for patients who require long-term enteral feeding and whose stomach is surgically absent or inaccessible. This population consists largely of those patients who have undergone surgical resection for the treatment of esophageal and or stomach cancer. Jejunostomy is also occasionally used for decompression of the jejunum. Rarely, jejunostomy is performed to facilitate biliary interventions in the setting of Roux-en-Y or other biliodigestive anastomoses [20].

Contraindications

Successful gastrostomy requires percutaneous access to the stomach and can therefore be hampered by interposition of other structures (e.g., liver, colon) or surgical alteration of the stomach. Generally, overlying left lobe of the liver is easily detected via ultrasound and is often remedied by insufflation of the stomach. An interposed colon, which does not displaced on inflation of the stomach, conveys significant risk for bowel perforation and secondary peritonitis. If a safe percutaneous access window cannot be identified on fluoroscopy, these cases often need gastrostomy placement under the guidance of cone-beam CT or conventional CT. Rarely, surgical gastrostomy is indicated in these cases.

Prior stomach surgery, especially gastrojejunal anastomosis and partial gastrectomies, can pose a challenge to fluoroscopic placement of PRG. In these cases, the stomach cannot often be sufficiently inflated with air for percutaneous puncture as there is no competent pyloric sphincter. Glucagon, which temporarily inhibits peristalsis, can be helpful in such cases prior to air insufflation. In difficult cases, the stomach may be accessible under cone-beam CT or regular CT guidance. Large hiatal hernias may present similar anatomical barriers to percutaneous gastrostomy, as there may be insufficient subdiaphragmatic stomach to permit safe access.

Patients with advanced cirrhosis often require supplemental nutrition, but the presence of ascites and esophageal or gastric varices can complicate or prevent the placement of percutaneous gastrostomies. The presence of gastric varices is a relative contraindication to percutaneous gastrostomy because of the risk of disruption of and subsequent hemorrhage from a gastric varix during puncture. Despite this risk, percutaneous gastrostomy has been successfully performed in patients with varices. The supplementation of fluoroscopy with ultrasound guidance to ensure the avoidance of varices during puncture has been utilized [21, 22]. Ascites conveys additional risks in patients undergoing gastrostomy but is not an absolute contraindication. The presence of ascites can make puncture more difficult, and a large amount of ascites between the stomach and abdominal wall increases the distance across the peritoneum that the catheter must traverse, leading to higher rates of tube dislodgment [19]. Ascites can be infected secondary to the procedure, and thus adequate gastropexy should be assured in these cases. Additionally, ascites can impair tract formation, necessitating paracentesis prior to and 7–10 days post procedure [23].

Patients with peritoneal carcinomatosis often develop malignant bowel obstruction. While venting gastrostomy may relieve such obstruction, the presence of peritoneal malignancy and frequently coexisting ascites can make percutaneous placement difficult. Tumor implantation in the peritoneum can directly obstruct puncture of the stomach or prevent adequate distention of the stomach to allow for safe puncture [19].

Gastrostomy placement may place patients with ventriculoperitoneal shunts at a theoretical risk of shunt infection and subsequent ventriculitis, meningitis, and encephalitis. Studies have found conflicting results as to whether gastrostomy placement increases the risk of shunt infection in practice [24–26].

Technique

Tube Selection

The indications for gastrostomy largely dictate the type of tube used (Table 3.2). Gastrostomy is usually sufficient for the purposes of venting in which decompression is the sole indication for stoma placement. Gastrostomy has some advantages over jejunal delivery of enteral feeds in that it may allow for nutritional supplementation in a way that better recreates normal oral feeding. Because the esophagus does not contribute significantly to digestion or absorption, gastric feeding can include a variety of feeds and bolus feeding. Jejunal feeding requires formed element feedings via a drip, which approximates the contents and rate of gastric emptying. Jejunostomy feedings cannot be given as boluses. Gastrojejunostomy (transgastric jejunostomy)

Table 3.2 Selection of procedure by indication

Procedure	Indication
Gastrostomy (Figs. 3.1, 3.2, and 3.3)	Enteral feeding, decompression
Gastrojejunostomy (transgastric jejunostomy) (Fig. 3.4)	Enteral feeding especially when the risk of reflux and aspiration is high
Dual-lumen gastrojejunostomy (Fig. 3.5).	Simultaneous jejunal feeding and gastric venting in gastric outlet obstruction
Direct jejunostomy	Enteral feeding in those cases in which the stomach cannot be accessed safely

is utilized for delivery of enteral feeds to the jejunum when the risk of aspiration from gastric delivery is felt to be high. Primary percutaneous jejunostomy is reserved as an option for enteral feeding in those cases in which puncture of the stomach is not feasible due to its absence or inaccessibility.

Preparation for Gastrostomy

The goals of patient preparation are to ensure the patient is informed and consents to the procedure and that the potential for complications is minimized. Coagulopathy must be screened for and corrected, the patient should fast to reduce the risk of aspiration, the stomach should be insufflated to facilitate entry, and the location of the colon and liver should be ascertained.

Though gastric bleeding occurs in only 1–3% of PRG or PEG procedures, precautions should be taken to ensure life-threatening hemorrhage does not occur. Gastric bleeding secondary to gastrostomy placement is less common with radiologically guided placements as compared to PEG and surgical methods [27].

Current consensus guidelines from the SIR recommend preprocedural testing of INR and aPTT and correction INR to less than 1.5. While severe thrombocytopenia can result in an increased bleeding risk with image-guided interventions, the relationship between thrombocytopenia and risk of clinically relevant bleeding varies with the etiology of thrombocytopenia and the presence of comorbidities. Thrombocytopenia caused by platelet consumption (i.e., ITP) is generally less likely to cause bleeding as compared to thrombocytopenia caused by decreased platelet production. In the presence of uremia, platelet function must be considered in addition to platelet number. It has been recommended by SIR consensus guidelines to have a platelet count of 40,000–50,000 μL prior to an invasive procedure [28].

Current consensus guidelines from the Society of Interventional Radiology recommend withholding clopidogrel for 5 days before gastrostomy tube placement but do not recommend withholding aspirin [28].

Oral administration of 200–300 mL of dilute barium approximately 12 h prior to the procedure is useful for delineation of the colon and to exclude the possibility of bowel obstruction. When time is limited, rectal administration of radiocontrast can be performed closer to the time of the procedure. Placement of a nasogastric tube is necessary for insufflation of the stomach with air prior to puncture. The stomach is usually distended with approximately 600 mL to a liter of room air. Glucagon administration (0.5–1 mg) prior to air insufflation helps to keep the pyloric valve closed and prevents dumping of air in the duodenum and small bowel. It is important that the stomach is well distended prior to puncture and tract dilatation. The risk of puncturing both gastric walls is increased when puncture is attempted in a non-distended stomach. With adequate insufflation of the stomach, the liver will likely not overlie the stomach, but verification of the liver margin via abdominal US can be performed prior to gastrostomy [18, 29, 30].

An intravenous line is required for the administration of sedation and analgesia. Intraprocedural cardiopulmonary monitoring should be used. A sterile field with appropriate draping and preparation should be maintained and the proposed area of puncture anesthetized with lidocaine. The utilization of preprocedural antibiotics varies by institution, but cefazolin is commonly administered in the immediate pre-procedural period. A clear benefit of prophylactic antibiotic administration has been demonstrated in patients undergoing gastrostomy placement in the setting of head and neck cancer [1].

Gastropexy

Gastropexy is a simple procedure by which the stomach is closely approximately to the internal abdominal wall to avoid or reduce leakage of catheter contents and stomach contents into the peritoneum and to reduce intraperitoneal migration of catheters. Simply, after stomach insufflation a 2×2 cm^2 is envisioned around the proposed puncture site. A 2×2 cm^2 should be demarcated around the area of proposed puncture and the corners of this square anesthetized with lidocaine. A T-fastener is then loaded onto a slotted needle and is inserted into the stomach, with verification of the position by air aspiration. A stylet is then used to deploy the T-fastener into the stomach, and mild tension on the suture approximates the stomach to the interior abdominal wall. The T-fastener's external fixation mechanism is then used to stabilize the T-fastener. The T-fastener sutures are then cut approximately 1–2 weeks after placement. T-fasteners with absorbable sutures are also commercially available.

The merits of performing of a gastropexy prior to gastrostomy are debated. Previously, several authors argued that the procedure is unnecessary, especially when utilizing smaller gauge catheters [31], however, in a prospective randomized trial demonstrated increased complication rates when gastropexy was not performed [32]. Variations on the technique exist across institutions and providers and methods with and without gastropexy are still being used [33–35].

Follow-Up

Following PRG placements, patients should be monitored for signs of peritonitis with serial abdominal exams. Many practices continue intermittent NG tube suction for the first 24 h to minimize the risk of gastric content leak. Feedings should not be immediately started after placement of PRG and clamping of the tube for at least 24 h post placement may be prudent in cases in which decompression is not required. If gastric decompression is necessary, the tube can be placed on intermittent suction immediately.

Patients and their caretakers should be counseled on the proper maintenance of their tubes and the possible complications they face. Flushing of the tube with 20 mL of water after each feeding and every 12 h is important to avoid clogging of the tube. The administration of crushed pills via the tube is inadvisable, and, if possible, pharmacists should be consulted to obtain elixir formulations of necessary medications.

Complications

Percutaneous radiologic gastrostomy is a relatively safe procedure. Major complications include infections, bleeding, and tube displacement. Infection secondary to radiologic gastrostomy can manifest as peritonitis, stomal infection, and sepsis. Peritonitis should be monitored for, as it requires prompt surgical attention. It occurs as a result of gastric contents leaking into the peritoneum due to insufficient gastropexy or due to leakage of gastric contents around the tube.

Stomal infections occur rarely, and prophylactic antibiotics have not been sufficiently shown to be useful. Owing to the oral/esophageal contact, PEG and peroral radiologic gastrostomy theoretically carry this elevated risk of stomal infection, and thus prophylactic antibiotics can be considered.

Chemical burns around G-tube site are the result of leakage of highly acidic stomach contents onto the skin. Persistence leakage and tenderness around the G-tube site is likely due to either tube clogging or secondary to underlying gastric outlet obstruction GOO (mechanical or vagal nerve dysfunction). Treatment options include skin care, regular tube flushing, exchange for larger G tube, GJ tube with decompression through G port or balloon dilatation, or stenting of the pylorus in suspected GOO.

A small pneumoperitoneum immediately after the procedure is normal. A large pneumoperitoneum, in the absence of symptoms, is usually of no clinical significance. However, cessation of tube feedings, antibiotics, and tightening the external bolster could help to resolve a large persistent pneumoperitoneum especially with concern for peritonitis.

Buried bumper syndrome represents a less common but serious complication of gastrostomy where the internal bumper retention erodes into the gastric wall causing ischemic necrosis and ultimate migration of the bumper between the gastric wall and the skin. Diagnosis is performed clinically (severe pain and erythema at tube site) and confirmed with endoscopy or CT scan. Treatment includes removal of the tube and the bumper, antibiotics, and placement of a new tube at a different site.

Clogging of the tube is a common occurrence and can be rectified by rigorous tube care. PRGs should be flushed with 20 mL of water after each use. Patient and caretaker education is essential to the avoidance of tube clogging.

Accidental dislodgement of the catheter is quite common and may be very painful. Once the tract has matured, replacement is relatively simple procedure as a new tube can be placed into the established tract under fluoroscopy.

References

1. Covarrubias DA, O'Connor OJ, McDermott S, Arellano RS. Radiologic percutaneous gastrostomy: review of potential complications and approach to managing the unexpected outcome. AJR Am J Roentgenol. 2013;200(4):921–31.
2. Ozmen MN, Akhan O. Percutaneous radiologic gastrostomy. Eur J Radiol. 2002;43(3):186–95.
3. Cozzi G, Gavazzi C, Civelli E, Milella M, Salvetti M, Scaperrotta G, et al. Percutaneous gastrostomy in oncologic patients: analysis of results and expansion of the indications. Abdom Imaging. 2000;25(3):239–42.
4. Laasch HU, Martin DF. Radiologic gastrostomy. Endoscopy. 2007;39(3):247–55.
5. James A, Kapur K, Hawthorne AB. Long-term outcome of percutaneous endoscopic gastrostomy feeding in patients with dysphagic stroke. Age Ageing. 1998;27(6):671–6.
6. George BP, Kelly AG, Albert GP, Hwang DY, Holloway RG. Timing of percutaneous endoscopic gastrostomy for acute ischemic stroke: an observational study from the US nationwide inpatient sample. Stroke. 2017;48(2):420–7.
7. Ho CS, Yeung EY. Percutaneous gastrostomy and transgastric jejunostomy. AJR Am J Roentgenol. 1992;158(2):251–7.
8. Righi PD, Reddy DK, Weisberger EC, Johnson MS, Trerotola SO, Radpour S, et al. Radiologic percutaneous gastrostomy: results in 56 patients with head and neck cancer. Laryngoscope. 1998;108(7):1020–4.
9. Tessier W, Piessen G, Briez N, Boschetto A, Sergent G, Mariette C. Percutaneous radiological gastrostomy in esophageal cancer patients: a feasible and safe access for nutritional support during multimodal therapy. Surg Endosc. 2013;27(2):633–41.
10. Thornton FJ, Fotheringham T, Alexander M, Hardiman O, McGrath FP, Lee MJ. Amyotrophic lateral sclerosis: enteral nutrition provision--endoscopic or radiologic gastrostomy? Radiology. 2002;224(3):713–7.
11. Montgomery ML, Miner NK, Soileau MJ, McDonald DK. Placement of the AbbVie PEG-J tube for the treatment of Parkinson's disease in the interventional radiology suite. Proc (Baylor Univ Med Cent). 2016;29(4):420–2.
12. Dhooge M, Gaudric M. Non-surgical access for enteral nutritional: gastrostomy and jejunostomy, technique and results. J Visc Surg. 2013;150(3 Suppl):S19–26.
13. Finucane TE, Christmas C. More caution about tube feeding. J Am Geriatr Soc. 2000;48(9):1167–8.
14. Lawinski M, Gradowski L, Bzikowska A, Goszczynska A, Jachnis A, Forysinski K. Gastrojejunostomy inserted through PEG (PEG-J) in prevention of aspiration pneumonia. Clinical nutrition complication in dysphagic patients. Pol Przegl Chir. 2014;86(5):223–9.
15. Anstee QM, Forbes A. The safe use of percutaneous gastrostomy for enteral nutrition in patients with Crohn's disease. Eur J Gastroenterol Hepatol. 2000;12(10):1089–93.
16. Sy K, Dipchand A, Atenafu E, Chait P, Bannister L, Temple M, et al. Safety and effectiveness of radiologic percutaneous gastrostomy and gastro jejunostomy in children with cardiac disease. AJR Am J Roentgenol. 2008;191(4):1169–74.
17. Laasch HU, Wilbraham L, Bullen K, Marriott A, Lawrance JA, Johnson RJ, et al. Gastrostomy insertion: comparing the options--PEG, RIG or PIG? Clin Radiol. 2003;58(5):398–405.
18. Lyon SM, Pascoe DM. Percutaneous gastrostomy and gastrojejunostomy. Semin Interv Radiol. 2004;21(3):181–9.
19. Shaw C, Bassett RL, Fox PS, Schmeler KM, Overman MJ, Wallace MJ, et al. Palliative venting gastrostomy in patients with malignant bowel obstruction and ascites. Ann Surg Oncol. 2013;20(2):497–505.
20. Overhagen H, Schipper J. Percutaneous jejunostomy. Semin Interv Radiol. 2004;21(3):199–204.
21. Horoldt BS, Lee FK, Gleeson D, McAlindon ME, Sanders DS. Ultrasound guidance in the placement of a percutaneous endoscopic gastrostomy (PEG): an adjuvant technique in patients with abdominal wall varices? Dig Liver Dis. 2005;37(9):709–12.

22. Kynci JA, Chodash HB, Tsang TK. PEG in a patient with ascites and varices. Gastrointest Endosc. 1995;42(1):100–1.
23. O'Connor OJ, Diver E, McDermott S, Covarrubias DA, Shelly MJ, Growdon W, et al. Palliative gastrostomy in the setting of voluminous ascites. J Palliat Med. 2014;17(7):811–21.
24. Gassas A, Kennedy J, Green G, Connolly B, Cohen J, Dag-Ellams U, et al. Risk of ventriculo-peritoneal shunt infections due to gastrostomy feeding tube insertion in pediatric patients with brain tumors. Pediatr Neurosurg. 2006;42(2):95–9.
25. Sane SS, Towbin A, Bergey EA, Kaye RD, Fitz CR, Albright L, et al. Percutaneous gastrostomy tube placement in patients with ventriculoperitoneal shunts. Pediatr Radiol. 1998;28(7):521–3.
26. Kim JS, Park YW, Kim HK, Cho YS, Kim SS, Youn NR, et al. Is percutaneous endoscopic gastrostomy tube placement safe in patients with ventriculoperitoneal shunts? World J Gastroenterol. 2009;15(25):3148–52.
27. Seo N, Shin JH, Ko GY, Yoon HK, Gwon DI, Kim JH, et al. Incidence and management of bleeding complications following percutaneous radiologic gastrostomy. Korean J Radiol. 2012;13(2):174–81.
28. Patel IJ, Davidson JC, Nikolic B, Salazar GM, Schwartzberg MS, Walker TG, et al. Consensus guidelines for periprocedural management of coagulation status and hemostasis risk in percutaneous image-guided interventions. J Vasc Interv Radiol. 2012;23(6):727–36.
29. Given MF, Hanson JJ, Lee MJ. Interventional radiology techniques for provision of enteral feeding. Cardiovasc Intervent Radiol. 2005;28(6):692–703.
30. Given MF, Lyon SM, Lee MJ. The role of the interventional radiologist in enteral alimentation. Eur Radiol. 2004;14(1):38–47.
31. Deutsch LS, Kannegieter L, Vanson DT, Miller DP, Brandon JC. Simplified percutaneous gastrostomy. Radiology. 1992;184(1):181–3.
32. Thornton FJ, Fotheringham T, Haslam PJ, McGrath FP, Keeling F, Lee MJ. Percutaneous radiologic gastrostomy with and without T-fastener gastropexy: a randomized comparison study. Cardiovasc Intervent Radiol. 2002;25(6):467–71.
33. Black MT, Hung CA, Loh C. Subcutaneous T-fastener gastropexy: a new technique. AJR Am J Roentgenol. 2013;200(5):1157–9.
34. Bendel EC, McKusick MA, Fleming CJ, Friese JL, A Woodrum D, Stockland AH, et al. Percutaneous radiologic gastrostomy catheter placement without gastropexy: a co-axial balloon technique and evaluation of safety and efficacy. Abdom Radiol (NY). 2016;41(11):2227–32.
35. Lyon SM, Haslam PJ, Duke DM, McGrath FP, Lee MJ. De novo placement of button gastrostomy catheters in an adult population: experience in 53 patients. J Vasc Interv Radiol. 2003;14(10):1283–9.

Chapter 4
Ascites Management

Michael Baldwin and Mark Amirault

Introduction

Ascites is defined as the pathologic accumulation of greater than 25 mL of fluid within the peritoneal cavity. Portal hypertension secondary to hepatic cirrhosis represents the cause of ascites in approximately 80% of patients in the United States [1]. Ascites is the most common complication of hepatic cirrhosis and develops in 35–50% of patients within 10 years of their initial diagnosis of cirrhosis [2].

The intraabdominal accumulation of ascites can result in disabling symptoms such as early satiety, malnutrition, fatigue, respiratory distress, and increased susceptibility to bacterial infections [3]. The development of ascites in patients with portal hypertension and cirrhosis is a poor prognostic indicator, with liver transplant-free mortality rates ranging from 15–20% at 1 year to 50–60% at 5 years from the first onset of ascites [4, 5]. Further, 10% of patients with cirrhosis develop refractory ascites, which portends substantial morbidity and mortality with a one-year survival of less than 50% [6].

Many other etiologies can also result in ascites, such as an underlying malignancy and heart failure, which represent the second and third most common causes of ascites in the United States, respectively (Table 4.1). Of note, approximately 5% of patients with ascites have more than one cause, such as cirrhosis plus peritoneal carcinomatosis, heart failure, and/or diabetic nephropathy [7].

M. Baldwin (✉)
University of Connecticut Health Center, Farmington, CT, USA
e-mail: mbaldwin@uchc.edu

M. Amirault
University of New England, Biddeford, Maine, USA

© Springer International Publishing Switzerland 2018
C. K. Singh (ed.), *Gastrointestinal Interventional Radiology*, Clinical Gastroenterology, https://doi.org/10.1007/978-3-319-91316-2_4

Table 4.1 Causes of ascites

Portal hypertension (84%)
Presinusoidal: portal vein thrombosis
Sinusoidal: cirrhosis, hepatitis, liver failure, vitamin A toxicity
Postsinusoidal: veno-occlusive disease, Budd-Chiari syndrome, constrictive pericarditis, congestive heart failure
Neoplasm (10%)
Peritoneal carcinomatosis
Lymphoma
Hepatocellular carcinoma
Ovarian carcinoma
Intra-abdominal mesothelioma
Inflammatory (3%)
Infectious process: tuberculosis, Whipple disease
Chemical causes: talc peritonitis
Immunologic disorder: systemic lupus erythematosus, vasculitides
Allergic causes: eosinophilic gastroenteritis
Miscellaneous (3%)
Hypoalbuminemia: nephrotic syndrome, protein-losing enteropathy, malnutrition
Diabetic nephropathy
Dialysis-associated ascites (nephrogenic ascites)
Ovarian hyperstimulation syndrome
Thoracic duct obstruction—chylous ascites

Adapted from Hou W, et al. [8] and Runyon BA, et al. [7]

Initial Diagnosis

The initial diagnosis of ascites is established with a combination of physical examination and abdominal imaging. Patients suspected of having ascites based on history and physical examination should undergo prompt abdominal imaging to confirm the presence of ascites and to evaluate for the presence of underlying hepatic cirrhosis and/or an intraabdominal malignancy.

Ultrasonography of the abdomen represents a rapid, cost-effective, and sensitive imaging method in the evaluation of ascites. Ultrasound can detect volumes of ascites as small as 5–10 mL [9]. Ultrasound evaluation also involves no exposure to ionizing radiation, requires no intravenous access, and does not represent an increased risk for contrast allergy and/or nephropathy.

Ultrasound, CT, or magnetic resonance imaging (MRI) can reveal evidence of a nodular, heterogeneous liver in patients with cirrhosis. In addition, ultrasound findings in patients with portal hypertension include dilation of the portal vein to ≥ 13 mm, dilation of the splenic and superior mesenteric veins to ≥ 11 mm, reduction in portal venous blood flow velocity, splenomegaly (diameter > 12 cm), and recanalization of the umbilical vein [10]. Follow-up hepatic MRI or CT of the abdomen and pelvis should be performed if the initial ultrasonographic examination demonstrates findings concerning for hepatocellular carcinoma or underlying intraabdominal malignancy.

The International Ascites Club has proposed a grading system of ascites. Grade 1 is mild ascites which is only detectable with ultrasound examination. Grade 2 or moderate ascites represents a volume of ascites that results in symmetric abdominal distention. Grade 3 ascites represents marked abdominal distention secondary to a large volume of ascites [11]. Of note, a positive shifting dullness on abdominal examination indicates the presence of approximately 1500 mL [12].

Diagnostic Paracentesis

Once the presence of ascites is established with physical examination and diagnostic imaging, the next clinical step is to determine the underlying etiology. Diagnostic paracentesis is recommended by the American Association for the Study of Liver Diseases (AASLD) at the time of a patient's initial presentation with ascites [13].

Ultrasound guidance can be used to locate ascitic fluid within the left or right lower quadrants of the abdomen, anterosuperior to the iliac crests. Care should be taken with color Doppler imaging to avoid the inferior epigastric vessels within the anterior abdominal wall when selecting the site of entry. One, 1.5, or 3.5 inch 22 gauge needles can be used with ultrasound guidance to obtain a small volume of ascitic fluid for laboratory analysis. Approximately 25 mL of ascites is needed for adequate initial laboratory evaluation of ascitic fluid that should include a cell count and differential, total protein and albumin, serum-ascites albumin gradient (SAAG), LDH, glucose, and specific gravity. If infection is suspected, ascitic fluid should also be inoculated in blood culture bottles prior to the initiation of antibiotics.

There are several generally accepted clinical indications for the performance of diagnostic abdominal paracentesis, in addition to the initial presentation of ascites (Table 4.2). Of note, prompt diagnostic paracentesis should be performed on the day of admission for a patient with preexisting ascites who is admitted to the hospital, regardless of the reason for the admission. Further, diagnostic paracentesis should be performed as soon as possible for a patient with ascites who demonstrates signs of clinical deterioration, such as fever, abdominal pain/tenderness, hepatic encephalopathy, peripheral leukocytosis, deterioration in renal function, or metabolic acidosis.

The performance of a diagnostic paracentesis on the day of admission to the hospital in a patient with cirrhosis and ascites has been demonstrated to decrease short-term mortality by 24% [14]. In addition to helping to clarify the cause of ascites and evaluating for potential infection, diagnostic paracentesis can identify unexpected diagnoses, such as chylous, hemorrhagic, or eosinophilic ascites.

Table 4.2 Indications for diagnostic paracentesis

Initial diagnosis of ascites
Each subsequent admission to the hospital (regardless of cause)
Clinical deterioration
Fever
Abdominal pain/tenderness
Mental status change
Ileus
Hypotension
Laboratory abnormalities
Peripheral leukocytosis
Acidosis
Decreasing renal function
Gastrointestinal hemorrhage (high risk for infection)

Abdominal paracentesis is essential in determining the cause of ascites and in evaluating for the presence of spontaneous bacterial peritonitis (SBP). SBP is defined by the presence of infected ascites in the absence of a surgically treatable intra-abdominal source in patients with cirrhosis. Ascitic fluid demonstrates $\geq$250/mm^3 polymorphonuclear cells [15].

SBP occurs in 10–30% of hospitalized cirrhotic patients with ascites regardless of the cause of admission [13]. Patients with SBP have an in-hospital mortality rate of 10% [16]. Of note, in-hospital mortality increases 3.3% in patients with SBP for every hour of delay in the performance of paracentesis [17].

The benefits of abdominal paracentesis in patients with appropriate indications almost always outweigh the risks of this routine procedure. Laboratory analysis of the ascitic fluid is vital in the determination of the cause(s) of the ascites and the presence of superimposed bacterial infection, and it can assist in the identification of antibiotic susceptibility of any organisms that are cultured.

Of note, patients do not have to be made NPO prior to paracentesis. In addition, an elevated international normalized ratio (INR) and thrombocytopenia are *not* contraindications to paracentesis, and in most patients there is no need to transfuse fresh frozen plasma or platelets prior to the procedure.

Seventy percent of patients with ascites have an abnormal prothrombin time, but the actual risk of bleeding following paracentesis is very low, with less than 1% of patients requiring a transfusion [18]. A prospective study of large-volume paracenteses documented no bleeding complications with no pre- or post-procedure transfusions despite INRs as high as 8.7 and platelet counts as low 19,000/mL [19].

Relative contraindications to paracentesis include disseminated intravascular coagulation and primary fibrinolysis. Patients with clinically apparent disseminated intravascular coagulation and oozing from needlesticks should be given platelets and, in some cases, fresh frozen plasma prior to the paracentesis. Paracentesis can be performed in patients with primary fibrinolysis, which should be suspected in patients with large, three-dimensional bruises, once treated with epsilon-aminocaproic acid [20].

Therapeutic Paracentesis

If the etiology of the patient's ascites is determined to be a result of hepatic cirrhosis, the patient should be evaluated for potential candidacy for liver transplantation. The patient should be immediately referred to a local liver transplantation center so that early evaluation can be initiated regardless of the model for end-stage liver disease (MELD) score at the time of referral.

In addition, all patients with initial presentation of ascites should be educated on proper restrictions of dietary sodium and, if they have concomitant hypervolemic hyponatremia, appropriate fluid restriction. The AASLD guidelines set forth dietary sodium restrictions as well as daily caloric intake goals and protein intake.

Initiation of diuretics is the first line of pharmacological therapy to assist dietary restrictions and promote an increase in fluid mobilization. Guidelines recommend starting an aldosterone antagonist initially, often spironolactone, to assist with diuresis. However, loop diuretics in combination, usually furosemide, can be used to enhance overall diuresis and net fluid removal [13].

If diuretic dose titration is unsuccessful, and other causes are excluded, patients with Grade 2 or 3 large-volume ascites may require intervention with serial large-volume paracentesis (LVP). Large-volume paracentesis is defined as the removal of ≥5 L of ascites. A 15 or 16 gauge paracentesis device can be used for LVP.

Paracentesis catheter drainage systems (Fig. 4.1) or sheathed centesis catheter needles (Fig. 4.2) with side holes can be advanced under sonographic visualization into the intra-abdominal ascites in order to remove large volumes of fluid. Vacuum bottles should be utilized to speed the removal of fluid.

Important postprocedure note: The AASD guidelines recommend administration of 6–8 g of intravenous albumin per liter of ascites drained during LVP in order to reduce the risk of circulatory dysfunction syndrome [13].

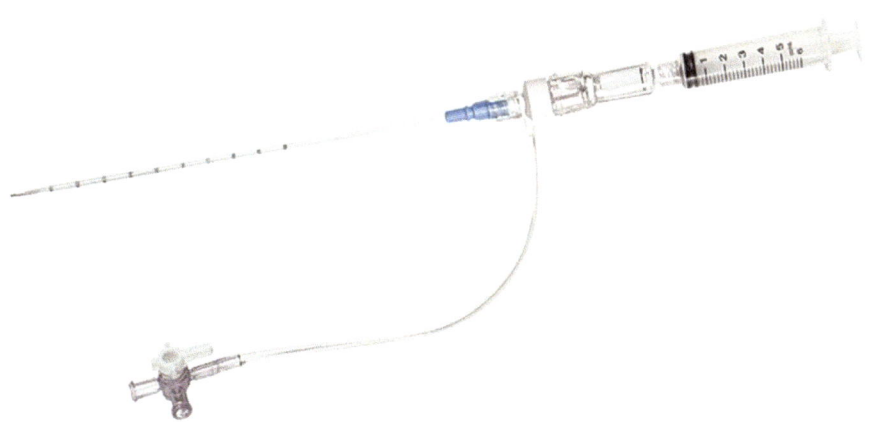

Fig. 4.1 Paracentesis catheter drainage system, *Safe-T-Centesis drainage system, Becton, Dickenson*

Fig. 4.2 Sheathed centesis
catheter needle, *Yueh
centesis catheter, Cook
Medical*

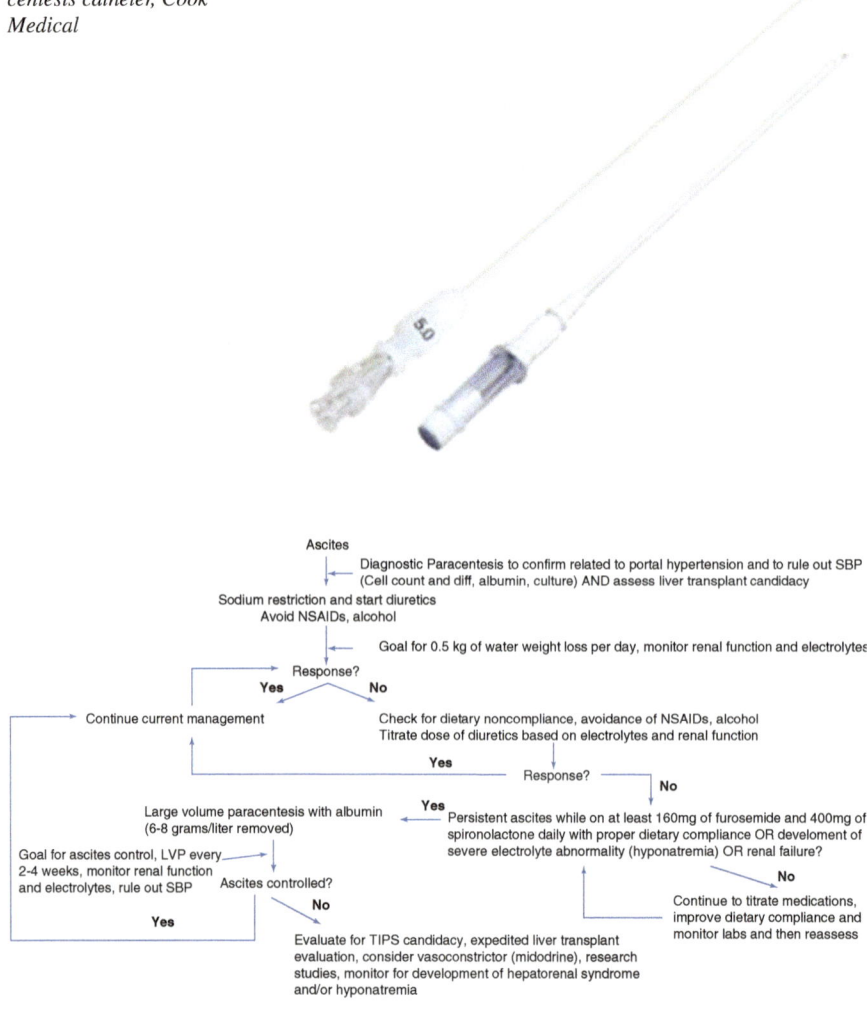

Fig. 4.3 An algorithm for the management of ascites and refractory ascites, *from Fortune* et al. [21]

If the patient requires more than two to three LVPs per month and can no longer tolerate or respond to maximum dose diuretics and dietary restrictions, the patient may have progressed to a more advanced stage of the liver disease with refractory ascites. In this case, the patient may need to be assessed for placement of a transjugular intrahepatic portosystemic shunt (TIPS) (Fig. 4.3).

Refractory Ascites

The effective arterial blood volume declines as liver disease progresses. Compensatory mechanisms involving the sympathetic nervous system and renal vasoconstriction attempt to improve blood volume, increasing plasma volume and increasing overall sodium and fluid retention. However, the loss of intravascular oncotic pressure secondary to hypoalbuminemia and increased intestinal capillary leakage lead to the eventual loss of effective blood volume maintenance.

These factors lead to severe renal vasoconstriction and impaired solute-free renal water excretion [22]. Thus, progressive hepatic disease can result in refractory ascites. Patients with refractory ascites demonstrate a lack of response to dietary management and medical treatment with rapid reaccumulation of ascites following LVP. Refractory ascites occurs in 10% of patients with cirrhosis and ascites [23].

Refractory ascites is associated with increased short-term mortality rates. Patients with refractory ascites demonstrate a 1-year mortality rate of near 70%, and over 50% of these patients will develop hepatorenal syndrome. Prompt evaluation for liver transplantation and/or TIPS should be performed for these patients [13].

Hepatic transplantation remains the only curative treatment of refractory ascites. Initial control of refractory ascites can be attempted with serial LVP with concomitant intravenous albumin administration. However, the effects are generally short lived with rapid reaccumulation of ascites.

Peritoneovenous shunts, such as the Denver shunt, are available (Fig. 4.4). These shunts allow the passage of ascitic fluid directly back into the central venous system.

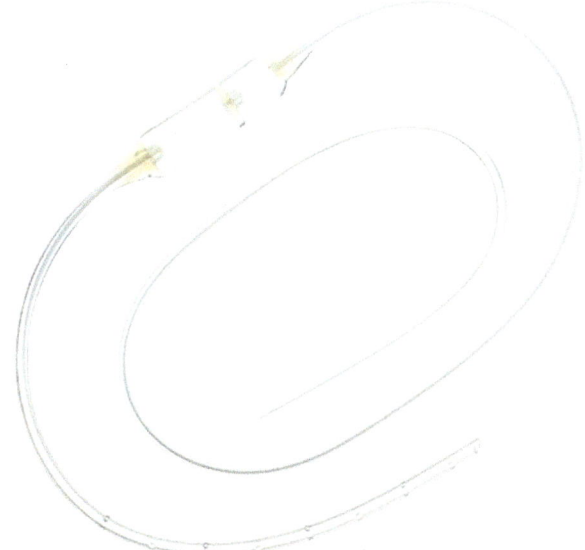

Fig. 4.4 Peritoneovenous shunt, *Denver shunt, Becton, Dickenson*

However, their use has declined in favor of TIPS due to associated complications [24]. Peritoneovenous shunts are associated with shunt occlusion, infection, post-shunt placement coagulopathy, deep venous thrombosis, and catheter breakage and leakage [25].

The placement of TIPS has resulted in improved control of ascites in patients with refractory ascites. Further, TIPS performed with polytetrafluoroethylene-covered (PTFE) stents results in improved transplant-free survival as well as ascites control without the major detriment of hepatic encephalopathy that was experienced with prior uncovered stents [26]. However, the prognosis of patients with refractory ascites remains grim; thus, referral to a liver transplantation centers remains critical for appropriate transplant candidates.

Patients with refractory ascites have increased risks of infection, especially SBP, as well as risk for further liver decompensation and hepatic encephalopathy, variceal hemorrhage, and risk of developing hepatorenal syndrome. Additional prospective studies are required to further elucidate optimal treatment management for these patients.

Malignant Ascites

Malignancy results in approximately 10% of cases of ascites [27]. Malignant ascites can develop secondary to gastric, colon, pancreatic, ovarian, endometrial, breast, lymphoma, and intra- abdominal mesothelioma. Approximately 10–15% of all patients with gastrointestinal malignancies developed ascites at some stage during their disease [28].

Malignant ascites is believed to occur secondary to at least four underlying mechanisms. Approximately 50% of cases are believed to develop secondary to peritoneal seeding, termed peripheral ascites. Chylous ascites is felt to account for approximately one fifth of cases, secondary to tumor invasion of the retroperitoneum resulting in lymphatic obstruction.

Hepatic metastases result in central ascites which is the most physiologically similar to ascites secondary to hepatic cirrhosis. Central ascites is believed to represent approximately 15% of malignant ascites cases. The remaining cases are felt to represent a combination of the above etiologies [29].

Most patients with malignant ascites have a poor prognosis with predictive survival of months. Medical management with diuretics and sodium restriction are not effective at decreasing malignant ascites. In addition, multiple clinic or hospital visits are required for serial LVP in many of these patients. Image-guided peritoneal drainage catheter placement has been shown to be a safe and effective management technique for the palliation of malignant ascites [30]. In addition, these catheters allow for the administration of intraperitoneal chemotherapy.

One such catheter, a PleurX catheter, is a cuffed tunneled drainage catheter that can be placed in the peritoneal cavity for the management of recurrent malignant

Fig. 4.5 PleurX peritoneal catheter drainage system, *Becton, Dickenson*

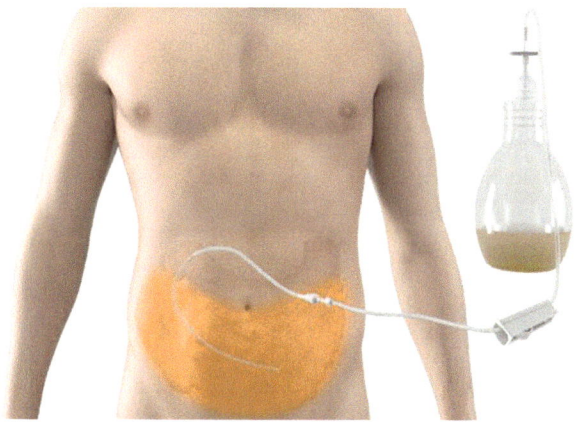

ascites (Fig. 4.5). These indwelling catheters have been demonstrated to be effective at relieving discomfort in patients with malignant ascites. Reported complications associated with PleurX catheters include ascites leakage, temporary weakness, catheter occlusion, peritonitis, and severe anemia due to bloody ascites [31]. However, these catheters allow patients to drain their malignant ascites in the comfort of their own homes and offer safe and effective palliation.

References

1. Runyon BA. Care of patients with ascites. N Engl J Med. 1994;330(5):337–42.
2. D'Amico G, Morabito A, Pagliaro L, Marubini E. Survival and prognostic indicators in compensated and decompensated cirrhosis. Dig Dis Sci. 1986;31(5):468–75.
3. Such J, Runyon BA. Spontaneous bacterial peritonitis. Clin Infect Dis. 1998;27(4):669–74.
4. Planas R, Montoliu S, Balleste B, et al. Natural history of patients hospitalized for management of cirrhotic ascites. Clin Gastroenterol Hepatol. 2006;4:1385–94.
5. D'Amico G, Garcia-Tsao G, Pagliaro L. Natural history and prognostic indicators of survival in cirrhosis: a systematic review of 118 studies. J Hepatol. 2006;44:217–31.
6. Arroyo V, Gines P. Planas 4. Treatment of ascites in cirrhosis. Diuretics, peritoneovenous shunt, and large volume paracentesis. Gastroenterol Clin N Am. 1992;21(1):237–56.
7. Runyon BA, Montano AA, Akriviadis EA, Antillon MR, Irving MA, McHutchison JG. The serum-ascites albumin gradient is superior to the exudate-transudate concept in the differential diagnosis of ascites. Ann Intern Med. 1992;117(3):215–20.
8. Hou W, Sanyal AJ. Ascites: diagnosis and management. Med Clin N Am. 2009;93:801–17.
9. Hanbridge AE, Lynch D, Wilson SR. US of the peritoneum. RadioGraphics. 2003;23:663–85.
10. Berzigotti A, Ashkenazi E, Reverter E, Abraldes JG, Bosch J. Non-invasive diagnostic and prognostic evaluation of liver cirrhosis and portal hypertension. Dis Markers. 2011;31(3):129–38.
11. Moore KP, Wong F, Gines P, Bernardi M, et al. The management of ascites in cirrhosis: report of the consensus conference of the International Ascites Club. Hepatology. 2003;38(1):258–66.
12. Runyon BA. Management of adult patients with ascites due to cirrhosis. Hepatology. 2004;39:1–16.

13. Runyon BA. Introduction to the revised American Association for the Study of Liver Diseases Practice Guideline Management of adult patients with ascites due to cirrhosis 2012. Hepatology. 2013;57(4):1651–3.
14. Orman ES, Hayashi PH, Bataller R, Barritt AS. Paracentesis is associated with reduced mortality in patients hospitalized with cirrhosis and ascites. Clin Gastroenterol Hepatol. 2014;12(3):496–503.
15. Runyon BA, Antillon MR. Ascitic fluid pH and lactate; insensitive and non-specific tests in detecting ascitic fluid infection. Hepatology. 1991;13:929–35.
16. Garcia-Tsao G. Spontaneous bacterial peritonitis: a historical perspective. J Hepatol. 2004;41:522–7.
17. Kim JJ, Tsukamoto DO, Mathur AK, Ghomri YM, Hou LA, et al. Delayed paracentesis in associated with increased in-hospital mortality in patients with spontaneous bacterial peritonitis. Am J Gastroenterol. 2014;109(9):1436–42.
18. Runyon BA. Paracentesis of ascitic fluid. A safe procedure. Arch Intern Med. 1986;146(11):2259–61.
19. Grabau CM, Grago SF, Hoff LK, Simon JA, et al. Performance standards for therapeutic abdominal paracentesis. Hepatology. 2004;40(2):484–8.
20. Gunawan B, Runyon BA. The efficacy and safety of epsilon-aminocaproic acid treatment in patients with cirrhosis and hyperfibrinolysis. Ailment Pharmacol Ther. 2006;23(1):115–20.
21. Fortune B, Cardenas A. Ascites, refractory ascites and hyponatremia in cirrhosis. Gastroenterol Rep. 2017;5(2):104–12.
22. Gines P, Cardenas A, Arroyo V, et al. Management of cirrhosis and ascites. N Engl J Med. 2004;350:1646–54.
23. Arroyo V, Gines P, Gerbes AL, et al. Definition and diagnostic criteria of refractory ascites and hepatorenal syndrome in cirrhosis; International Ascites Club. Hepatology. 1996;23:164–76.
24. Gines P, Arroyo V, Vargas V, et al. Paracentesis with intravenous infusion of albumin as compared with peritoneovenous shunting in cirrhosis with refractory ascites. N Engl J Med. 1991;325:829–35.
25. Martin LG. Percutaneous placement and management of peritoneovenous shunts. Semin Intervent Radiol. 2012;29(2):129–34.
26. Bureau C, Thabut D, Oberti F, et al. Transjugular intra hepatic portosystemic shunts with covered stents increase transplant-free survival of patients with cirrhosis and recurrent ascites. Gastroenterology. 2017;152:157–63.
27. Parsons SL, Watson SA, Steele RJC. Malignant ascites. Br J Surg. 1996;83:6–14.
28. Rosenberg SM. Palliation of malignant ascites. Gastroenterol Clin North Am. 2006;35:189–99.
29. Husbands EL. Targeting diuretic use for malignant ascites-two case reports highlighting the value of the serum-ascites albumin gradient in a palliative setting. J Pain Symptom Manag. 2010;39(2):e7-e9.
30. Akinci D, Erol B, Ciftci TT, Akhan O. Radiologically placed tunneled peritoneal catheter in palliation of malignant ascites. Eur J Radiol. 2011;80:265–8.
31. Courtney A, Nemcek AA, Rosenberg S, et al. Prospective evaluation of the PleurX catheter when used to treat recurrent ascites associated with malignancy. J Vasc Interv Radiol. 2008;19:1723–31.

Chapter 5
Abscess Drainage/Biopsy

Prasoon P. Mohan and Adam Swersky

Percutaneous Abdominal Abscess Drainage

Introduction

Percutaneous image-guided drainage has been firmly established as a primary treatment option for fluid collections in the abdomen and pelvis [1–3]. Minimally invasive image-guided drainage techniques have revolutionized the management of abdominal abscesses as in the past these cases often necessitated open surgical drainage. The minimally invasive nature of and the lower morbidity and mortality associated with percutaneous drainage make it the treatment of choice for the management of abscesses, hematomas, lymphoceles, bilomas, and any other type of intra-abdominal fluid collection. Specific indications and methods of percutaneous drainage for various pathologies will be discussed in the sections ahead.

Indications

Percutaneous drainage is indicated primarily for treatment of intra-abdominal abscesses, wherein the pus can be drained with catheters and samples obtained for culture and sensitivity to guide antibiotic therapies. Drainage of pus results in an

P. P. Mohan (✉)
Department of Vascular and Interventional Radiology, University of Miami - Miller School of Medicine, Jackson Memorial Hospital, Miami, FL, USA
e-mail: PXP136@med.miami.edu

A. Swersky
University of Miami Miller School of Medicine, Miami, FL, USA

© Springer International Publishing Switzerland 2018
C. K. Singh (ed.), *Gastrointestinal Interventional Radiology*, Clinical Gastroenterology, https://doi.org/10.1007/978-3-319-91316-2_5

instant reduction of pressure within the abscess cavity, leading to pain relief. Percutaneous drainage methods may also be used in the treatment of hematomas, lymphoceles, or other intra-abdominal located collections.

Contraindications

Absolute contraindications to percutaneous drainage of an abdominal collection include lack of a safe pathway to the lesion from interposed bowel, blood vessels, or otherwise significant viscera and uncorrectable coagulopathies. Any procedure requiring pleural transgression is relatively contraindicated due to the risks of pneumothorax, effusion, and empyema development. Sterile collections that have the potential to become secondarily infected following catheter drainage is a relative contraindication. Tumor abscess drainage is relatively contraindicated due to risk of tumor spread along the track and subsequent requirement for lifelong drainage.

Preprocedure Preparation

The patient should be counselled appropriately about the reason for the procedure and its risks, benefits, and alternatives. Capacity for consent should be assessed, as well as consideration of the need for anesthesiology consult. The patient should be instructed to be nil per oral for 6 h prior to the procedure. The patient should be instructed to arrive 1 h prior to the procedure, with proper arrangements made for transport (adult chaperone to transport to and from after conscious sedation).

Preprocedural Management of Anticoagulation/Labs

General recommendations for management of coagulation status are based on the SIR Standards of Practice consensus guidelines [4]. Percutaneous abdominal drainage (and biopsy) procedures are classified as procedures with moderate risk of bleeding [4]. Preprocedure laboratory testing should include serum INR <1.5 and platelets <50,000 μL. Aspirin need not be withheld for percutaneous drainages. Clopidogrel should be withheld for 5 days prior to procedure. Patients on therapeutic dose of low-molecular-weight heparin (LMWH) should only be advised to withhold one dose prior to the procedure (12 h).

IV access should be established using a 20-gauge needle or larger prior to procedure. Prophylactic antibiotics should be administered as determined by any blood cultures, or broad spectrum antibiotics should be used as recommended by local infectious disease protocol, although patients who are referred to IR for percutaneous abscess drainage are often already receiving antibiotic therapy [5]. Routine prophylaxis is recommended to cover for *S. aureus*, *S. epidermidis*, *Corynebacterium* spp., aerobic Gram-negative bacteria, and anaerobes [6]. Intra-abdominal abscesses most commonly contain Gram-negative rods such as *E. coli*, *Bacteroides fragilis*, and *Enterococcus* spp. [5, 7, 8]. Current antibiotic regimes involve the use of second- or third-generation cephalosporins, ampicillin/sulbactam, or a combination of clindamycin and gentamycin if the patient is severely allergic to penicillin [6, 9]. Please refer to the SIR Standards of Practice guidelines for adult antibiotic prophylaxis for more detailed information [6]. The use of prophylactic and/or broad spectrum antibiotics will not interfere with the results of drainage. Most procedures are done under moderate (conscious) sedation and local anesthesia. General anesthesia should be considered in young children, uncooperative patients, or patients with other significant comorbidities.

Imaging Modalities

Choice of imaging modality is extremely important for success of percutaneous drainage. Use of ultrasound (US) allows for real-time visualization of the collection, surrounding structures, and the needle or catheter. Real-time guidance is particularly valuable for collections that move with respiration or those which are in close proximity to the lung, bowel, or vasculature. The color Doppler feature of US can help differentiate between fluid collections and vascular malformations, which are extremely important to discern before drainage. US also provides the ability for doing bedside procedures. Limitations of US include cases in which visualization is impacted by body habitus, bone and bowel gas, or gas within the abscess.

Computed tomography (CT) is the most preferred modality for image guidance because it provides the most accurate visualization of anatomy and of the fluid collection. CT also allows for easy, optimal planning of the access route. To aid in the visualization of the abscess (compared to surrounding bowel), bowel opacification with Gastrografin can be used. Limitations of CT include lack of real-time guidance and difficulty in identifying loculations (when the septa have the same density as the adjacent fluid). It is especially useful to combine both US and CT guidance when real-time visualization is necessary. This can significantly increase the speed and safety of the procedure.

Technique

It is first and foremost important to review any prior imaging to visualize the abnormality and then decide on the appropriate guidance method, the route needed for drainage, and positioning of the patient. The patient should be clearly instructed regarding specific breathing techniques that might be necessary during the procedure. The initial CT should be performed with the patient in optimal position (supine, prone, or lateral decubitus—the latter of which may reduce risk of pleural transgression by splinting the ipsilateral hemithorax), and a radiopaque grid should be placed over the skin surface ideally with the patient's arms positioned overhead (to improve image quality). 5–10 mm slices are then taken through the region of interest. This planning scan should clearly reveal a safe route for skin puncture, needle angle, drainage route, and the distance to collection. Angling the gantry or changing the patient position may help if some of these metrics are not at first obvious.

A wide area surrounding the chosen entry site should then be sterilized and local anesthesia applied to the skin and soft tissue. Generally, the shortest possible distance without transgressing vital structures should be considered for the approach. Consider the size and shape of the abscess, and preferably use an extraperitoneal approach to avoid peritoneal contamination. During fine needle aspiration (FNA), it is permissible to traverse the liver, kidney, stomach, and small bowel but should be avoided in catheter drainage. Colonic loops and the pancreas should be especially avoided because of the risk of superinfection and pancreatitis, respectively. For pelvic abscesses, the anterior approach may prove difficult so transgluteal, transvaginal, or transrectal approaches should be considered and will be described in greater detail. Organ displacement techniques may also prove useful to create a better route for drainage or aspiration.

Initial aspiration of the fluid through a Yueh needle is used to determine quickly if a collection is infected or sterile prior to catheter placement. No more than a few milliliters are aspirated to prevent the cavity from collapsing.

The fluid aspirate can be inspected macroscopically for color, smell, viscosity, and turbidity. If the fluid is determined to be purulent, catheter placement is indicated. Fluid sample should be sent for gram stain, culture, and sensitivity. Following aspiration, if the needle is determined to be in good position, it may be used as a guide to place a catheter using the trocar technique or be used for the introduction of a guidewire for the Seldinger technique.

The technique for drainage (trocar vs. Seldinger) chosen by the interventional radiologist is determined based on the size of the collection, its location, the type of imaging guidance used, and the preference/experience. Generally, Seldinger technique is considered to be safer and is the more commonly used approach. Larger, more superficial collections are amenable to the trocar technique. Following needle access, a guidewire is passed into the collection, and the track is serially dilated using Teflon dilators. This is followed by introduction over the wire of the appropriately sized drainage catheter into the collection. It is important to take measures to avoid guidewire kinking, loss of access, and malposition during the procedure. Catheters employed in this manner may range in size from 7 to 14 Fr. Larger collections (and those with more viscous fluid) will require larger catheters (such as 12–14 Fr.). Alternatively, multi-side-hole catheters coiled over the length of the collection may prove to be an excellent option for spread-out or longitudinal collections. In the trocar technique, the whole catheter containing a sharp stylet is introduced into the collection under image guidance, often inserted adjacent and parallel to a reference needle placed into the collection.

Once the catheter is positioned within the cavity, it should be attached at the back end to a drainage bag via a three-way stopcock, which will allow for aspiration and irrigation of the area in a controlled manner. Aspiration should continue from the cavity until it is completely evacuated, as evidenced by absence of fluid return. Next, the cavity is irrigated with small aliquots of saline (5–20 mL) not exceeding the original volume aspirated (to avoid over-distending the cavity which may lead to bacteremia and sepsis). Irrigation should continue until the aspirate is clear or blood-tinged. US or CT imaging immediately following drainage will help in confirming the drainage of the entire cavity, detect any additional collections, and serve as a screening modality for complications (i.e., hemorrhage). Internally, the catheter should be secured using the locking loop. Externally, it should be secured by either suturing to the skin or by employing a commercially available fixation device.

In the drainage of hepatic abscesses (Fig. 5.1a–c), it is most important to avoid transgression of any of the large vessels, dilated bile ducts, and the gallbladder. Similarly, it is important to avoid transgression of the pleura if possible, which may be aided by adoption of an anterior and subcostal approach under a combination of US and CT guidance. Pyogenic abscesses are the most common liver collections that may be drained percutaneously as first-line treatment [10]. For echinococcal (hydatid) cysts, medical therapy is considered first-line treatment, and percutaneous drainage may be considered in those who have undergone at least 2 weeks of medical therapy [2]. In such cases, preparations should be made to treat potential anaphylaxis prior to treatment. Hypertonic saline should replace small aspirates taken prior to catheter placement to prevent leakage into the peritoneum and subsequent anaphylaxis. Similarly, amebic abscesses warrant medical therapy as first-line treatment, and in refractory cases or peripheral collections that are at risk of rupture drainage, it may be required [11]. Bilomas may be drained especially if they are superinfected and symptomatic. Splenic collections may be drained if coagulopathies have been corrected, and care is taken to avoid transgression of as much parenchyma as possible.

Percutaneous drainage is indicated for pancreatic pseudocysts if they are symptomatic (pain, obstruction of the biliary and/or GI tract), large in size (>5 cm), and suspected to be infected or if they have enlarged over time. Management of pancreatic abscesses (Fig. 5.2a, b) is challenging due to concurrent pancreatitis, systemic illness, their multiloculated nature, high viscosity, and the presence of particulate

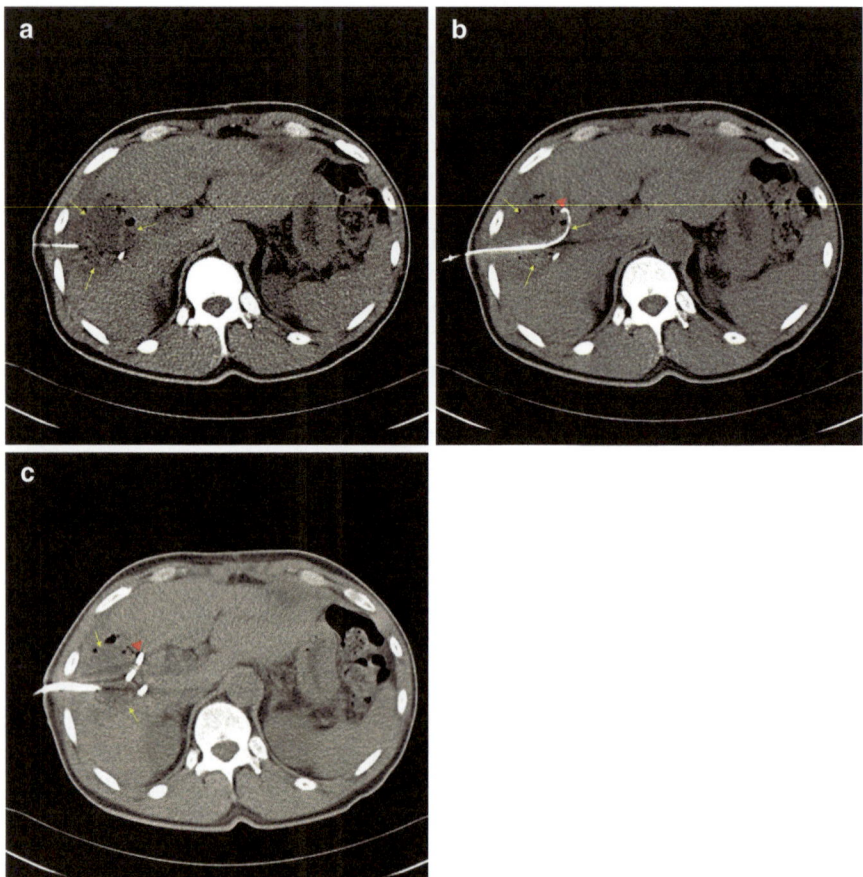

Fig. 5.1 (**a**) Liver abscesses (yellow arrows) are indicated for percutaneous drainage under CT guidance. (**b**) Per the Seldinger technique, a guidewire (red arrowhead) is used to access the collection (yellow arrows). (**c**) An APDL catheter (red arrowhead) within the collection (yellow arrows) is shown on CT

material which causes frequent catheter clogging. Larger catheters (14 to 26 Fr.) are indicated for these abscesses, and they require frequent lavage and catheter exchange due to clogging. Output that persists from the catheter over a prolonged period of time is suggestive of pancreatic fistula which can be confirmed with contrast injection of the catheter. Infusion of octreotide may be helpful in closing the pancreatic fistula. Percutaneous drainage under CT guidance is also indicated for infected pancreatic necrosis. This method may be curative in many cases despite a common notion that percutaneous drainage of these collections serves only as a bridge to surgery [12]. These collections need frequent catheter exchange and lavage and require prolonged drainage with larger catheters due to propensity for clogging.

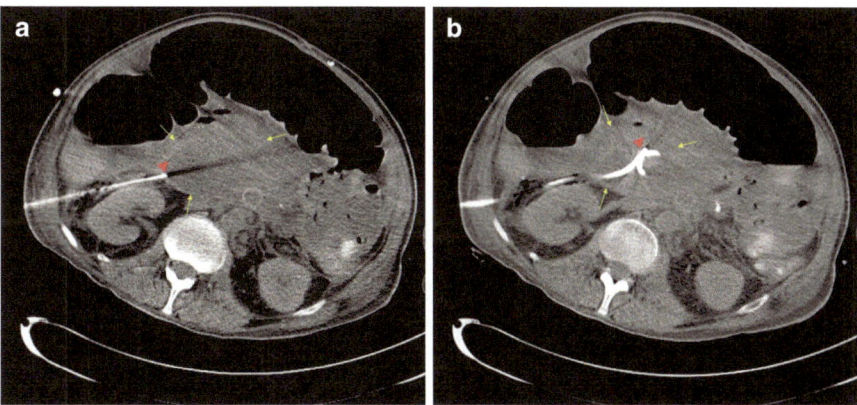

Fig. 5.2 (**a**) A peripancreatic abscess (marked by the yellow arrows) is indicated for percutaneous drainage under CT guidance. A Yueh needle (red arrowhead) is shown advancing into the collection. It is important to obtain images such as this one with confirmation of the needle tip within the collection. (**b**) An APDL catheter (red arrowhead) is shown in the peripancreatic abscess (yellow arrows)

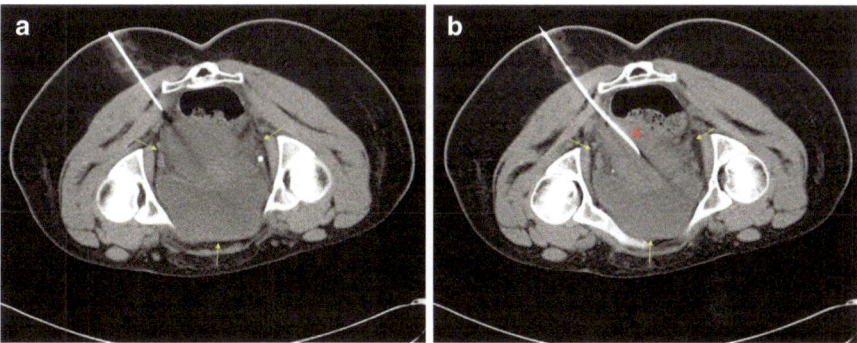

Fig. 5.3 (**a**) Pelvic abscesses, such as the one shown here (yellow arrows), are amenable to percutaneous drainage under CT guidance. (**b**) The pelvic abscess (yellow arrows) is accessed (red arrowhead)

Transgluteal drainage may be indicated in drainage of pelvic collections (Fig. 5.3a, b) [13]. The catheter should be inserted adjacent to the sacrococcygeal margin and below the piriformis muscle at the level of the sacrospinous ligament. It is important to follow this anatomic protocol in order to avoid neurovascular structures in the region, which includes the sacral plexus and inferior gluteal vessels. The vasculature needs to be clearly defined on the planning CT scan. Angling of the gantry can be very helpful in these cases. Transrectal drainage may be required when collections are anterior or posterior to the rectum and is included in the possible management of prostatic abscesses [14]. The patient should be placed in the lateral decubitus position for transrectal drainage procedures.

Postprocedure Management

Much of the postprocedure management revolves around care of the catheter, and it is essential that the care in this scenario is provided by the interventional radiologist and not offloaded to another member of the medical team. Daily inpatient rounds present an opportunity for the members of the interventional radiology team to see the patient and assess the outcomes of treatment. Irrigation of the catheter should occur every 8 h to prevent the catheter from occluding. Especially viscous collections may require more frequent drainage. Each time the catheter is flushed, 5 mL saline should be directed toward the collection, and 5 mL saline should be directed toward the bag. Suction is not necessary with the use of equally effective gravity drainage. Catheter removal can be considered once there is clinical improvement (fever and pain resolution, appearance, appetite) and vital signs and laboratory signs (i.e., white cell count) have normalized. It is essential that the catheter is not removed prematurely, as the collection can reaccumulate. Conversely, there is an associated increase in morbidity if the catheter is permitted to remain too long. Normalizing vital and laboratory signs is usually associated with catheter drainage of under 20 mL/day, which is another criteria warranting consideration for catheter removal.

Repeat imaging is generally unnecessary and should only be done if the patient is not improving clinically, if drainage is occurring at a lower rate than expected, or if there is an abrupt reduction in drainage. In this case, CT is preferred to visualize the anatomy of the collection and surrounding areas. If imaging reveals disappearance of the collection, this supports catheter removal as well. High output from the catheter, defined as greater than 50 mL/day (after the 4th day of insertion), indicates the possibility of bowel, pancreatic duct, or biliary fistula, and these possibilities must be investigated with abscessogram (injection of contrast through the catheter, Fig. 5.4). If a fistula is determined to exist, it should be promptly addressed, and the catheter may be needed to be left in for 4–6 weeks. In the specific case of pancreatic fistula, octreotide can be an adjunctive treatment. In the opposite case of low catheter output due to a highly viscous collection, 4–6 mg tissue plasminogen activator (tPA) diluted in 50 mL normal saline has proven to be a highly useful adjunct if used twice per day for 3 days (if this injected volume does not exceed the volume of the collection) [15]. The catheter should be clamped for 30 min after the tPA injection and then should be aspirated.

Results

Generally, percutaneous abdominal abscess drainage has a high success rate of 90% or greater [1, 16]. Percutaneous drainage for the treatment of infected pancreatic necrosis has been shown to have an estimated success rate of 84% in the most recent

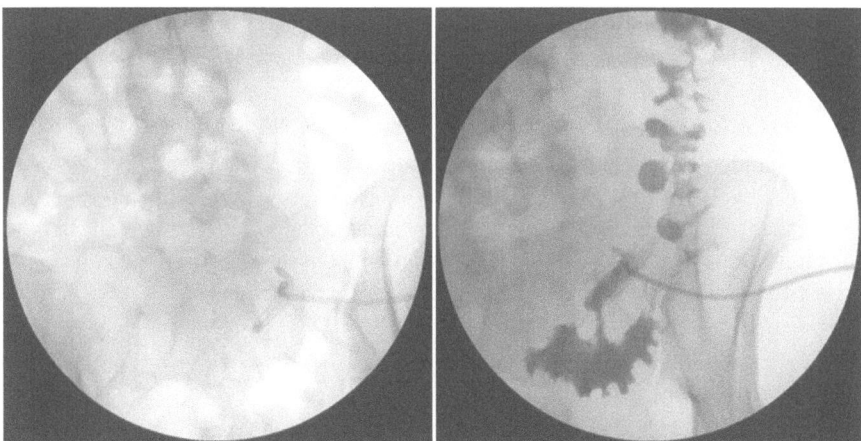

Fig. 5.4 *Abscessogram.* The patient has an indwelling pigtail catheter for abscess following laparotomy for perforated appendix. Catheter check demonstrates fistula to sigmoid colon. The catheter will have to stay longer for fistula to heal and for enterocutaneous track to mature

large study and has shown far lower morbidity (7%) as compared to surgical drainage (up to 78%) [17–19]. Recurrence of abscess can be expected to occur due to early catheter removal and fistula formation (undetected) or if the collection drained is a tumor abscess. Rate of recurrence ranges from 8 to 20% [2].

Complications

Complications from percutaneous abdominal abscess drainage occur in an estimated 10–15% of cases [1, 20]. Thirty-day mortality estimates range from 1 to 6%. Major complications from percutaneous abdominal abscess drainage include hemorrhage, perforation of the bladder or bowel, hemopneumothorax, septic shock, and peritonitis [3]. Blood vessel puncture can result in rapid hemorrhage and requires prompt angiographic intervention. Perforation can occur from direct trauma during catheter insertion. Should bowel injury be suspected, surgical consultation should direct the best management course. Septicemia is not uncommon at the time of drainage, occurring in 1–2% of cases [1]. Aggressive airway control, venous access, and resuscitative therapy comprising reperfusion with fluids and early antibiotic administration are all important steps in management [21, 22]. Minor complications may result as well, such as pain, bleeding, infection, and pericatheter leak [2]. Issues related to the catheter usually result from kinking, blocking, or movement of the catheter. These issues can be avoided with meticulous procedural technique and with monitoring of the catheter through daily flushing and aspiration.

Percutaneous Abdominal Biopsy

Introduction

Image-guided percutaneous abdominal biopsy is a minimally invasive technique that has revolutionized the evaluation of solitary masses, both deep and superficial [3]. It has replaced exploratory laparotomy and has led to reduced overall costs and complications [2, 23]. Percutaneous abdominal biopsy under image guidance is the most common interventional radiologic procedure performed.

Indications

Percutaneous abdominal biopsy is indicated in several scenarios [24]. Biopsy is essential in the diagnosis of primary neoplasm, verification of metastatic lesions, and staging. More recently, molecular and genetic analyses can be made using biopsy samples. Progression or regression of disease may be noted through chrono-logical analysis of biopsy specimens by a pathologist. Infectious and inflammatory diseases may be confirmed via biopsy.

Contraindications

Contraindications to percutaneous abdominal biopsy are essentially the same as for percutaneous abdominal drainage. Please refer to the prior section for details.

Preprocedure Preparation

Preprocedure preparation for percutaneous abdominal biopsy is essentially the same as in percutaneous abdominal drainage, aside from a few key differences high-lighted below. Please refer to the prior section for other details. This includes spe-cific anticoagulation management, which can also be found in the SIR Standards of Practice consensus guidelines [4].

In the case of adrenal mass biopsy where pheochromocytoma is part of the dif-ferential diagnosis, plasma-free fractionated metanephrines should be obtained due to high sensitivity, followed by measurement of 24-h urine-fractionated metaneph-rines and catecholamines to increase specificity [25]. It is highly recommended to arrange for a cytopathologist to be present during the biopsy procedure [26]. This will offer real-time assessment of the sample obtained and thus improves the yield. Should the sample be insufficient for any reason as determined by the cytopathologist, alternate approaches or repeat biopsy can be performed while still minimizing time for procedure and patient exposure to sedative, multiple needle passes or radiation. Additionally, special procedures that may need to be employed for adequate tissue sampling can occur on-site (i.e., biomarkers, electron microscopy, culture, etc.).

Preprocedural Management of Anticoagulation/Labs

Anticoagulation management for percutaneous abdominal biopsy is identical to that of percutaneous abdominal drainage. Please refer to the prior section for details.

Antibiotic prophylaxis for percutaneous biopsy is not recommended routinely, with the exception of biopsies performed transrectally [8]. Please refer to the SIR Standards of Practice guidelines for adult antibiotic prophylaxis for more detailed information [6].

Imaging Modalities

Choice of imaging modality is one of the essential first steps in planning a percutaneous abdominal biopsy procedure [23, 27]. Please refer to the prior section on percutaneous abdominal drainage for details on the benefits and drawbacks of each modality. Key differences for biopsy procedures are discussed here.

Fluoroscopy is used for transjugular biopsy of liver parenchyma. Deeply located, smaller lesions may not be visible on US and thus should be performed under CT guidance. In order to reduce needle placement time, continuous CT scanning may be used as well as the "quick check" method in which intermittent image capturing is alternated with increasingly accurate advancement of the needle toward the area of interest. MRI may also be used and should be considered when lesions have only been seen on MRI scans. MRI offers multi-planarity and does not subject the patient to ionizing radiation. Limitations to MRI usage include cost and limited availability.

Technique [27]

Please refer to the prior section on patient preparation in percutaneous abdominal drainage, as it is very similar to that of percutaneous abdominal biopsy. Key differences are included here.

If performing CT-guided biopsy, please refer to the prior section on percutaneous abdominal drainage for description on planning the route and optimizing patient positioning.

The skin and subcutaneous tissue layers should be anesthetized with 1–2% lidocaine and 3–5-mm incision made superficially with a scalpel. Next, the biopsy needle should be chosen. Sizes may range from fine (20–25-gauge) to large (14–19-gauge) and have varying roles. Finer needles should be reserved for cytology and cases in which bowel or pleura may be transgressed, because they are associated with lower hemorrhagic potential. Deeper lesions may require 20-gauge or larger due to their increased stiffness—needles smaller than this have a tendency to bend out of the needle track. Larger needles can be used for cytologic or histologic purposes and generally increase the yield of the sample. This allows for greater tissue subtyping (i.e., lymphoma—although smaller needles may be adequate) although it may increase hemorrhage risk. Needles may vary in the mechanism of cutting. End-cutting needles include acute bevel and 90° bevel, while side-cutting needles include cannula gap and stylet gap and may be spring-loaded (automated). When choosing the needle, it is important to consider lesion size, depth, route, suspected diagnosis, and cytopathologist preference. Cytopathologists often prefer a "cell-layer thick" sample, so finer needles may be preferred unless more sample is needed. In general, the thinnest needle that can be successfully employed for reaching the lesion and obtaining sample should be the one selected. In general, the shortest path to the lesion possible should be exercised and the safest instrument used, with the least number of needle placements. For lesions that move with respiration, a breath hold will be required for needle placement (preferably at end-expiration). The patient should practice before the procedure to maximize consistency. It is crucial to avoid transgressing certain structures during the needle placement, most notably the lungs, gallbladder, pancreas, dilated pancreatic or biliary ducts, and bowel loops (unless necessary—with a fine needle).

The coaxial method is very helpful when the need for precision is greater with smaller, deeper lesions. First, a biopsy cannula is placed into the lesion under image guidance. This reference needle may be simply an introducer needle or may be a biopsy needle. The size of the cannula must be able to accommodate the sampling needle. To use an 18-gauge side-cutting needle for specimen retrieval, a 17-gauge cannula is needed. A 20-gauge side-cutting needle requires a 19-gauge cannula. A 22-gauge end-cutting requires a 19-gauge (or larger) cannula. To sample the specimen using fine needle aspiration, small motions of the needle in an up-and-down and rotational fashion of the needle should accompany continuous suction (3–10 mL) with a 10-mL syringe connected by extension tubing. If the lesion is vascular, less suction (1–2 mL) is indicated. The most optimal portion of the lesion should always be targeted. Prior to the needle being removed from the lesion, the suction should be removed to prevent re-aspiration of contents. Automatic spring-loaded devices can be used to extract core tissue samples.

For US-guided biopsies, when the needle tip is in the lesion, it is important to capture this image in two views, with the transducer either perpendicular to the entry site or in the vicinity of the entry site. The ultrasound waves should travel parallel to the needle, which may be added by "bobbing" the needle up and down for aid in visualization. Many needles have echogenic tips that allow for clear visualization during scanning.

Cytology smears should be obtained dry. A cytopathologist present can aid in the processing of the specimen and check the adequacy of the sample. Core biopsy samples should be submitted in formalin solution to allow for proper histologic evaluation. If lymphoma is a possibility, the sample should be submitted in saline solution. Gram stains or cultures may also be warranted depending on the pathology. Certain technical maneuvers may aid in success during the biopsy procedure [2, 23, 28–31]. Hydrodissection of the planned needle track using sterile saline, contrast, or dextrose solution may help displacement of various structures. In the coaxial technique, a manually curved 22-gauge needle advanced through a large reference needle may help target a mass not precisely in line with the first reference needle. Contrast-enhanced CT may be necessary to delineate the anatomy. Newer technology such as electromagnetic tracking by means of skin fiducials combined with needles that have internal sensors can aid in the tracking of the needle tip in CT- or US-guided procedures. The triangulation method can be used in order to mathematically determine the ideal needle angle and distance to the target lesion. To maintain the needle in the imaging plane, the gantry tilt technique may be used as well. Embolization of the needle track through the cannula upon removal (to help reduce bleeding) may be attempted, with either an absorbable gelatin slurry (Gelfoam, Pfizer, New York, NY) or polyvinyl alcohol foam (Ivalon, Unipoint Lab, High Point, NC). Additionally, the stylet in coaxial technique may be inserted halfway and left to promote clot formation for 1–2 min and then injected into the track by advancing the stylet forward prior to removal.

Organ-Specific Biopsies of Focal Masses [2, 3, 11, 23, 29, 32–35]

For liver biopsy use of CT or US guidance will suffice. It is important to interrupt the liver "cuff," going transparenchymally to prevent bleeding into the peritoneum. For the adrenal gland, CT is the preferred modality unless the lesion is large enough to allow for visualization on US. For the adrenal gland, care should be taken to avoid transgression of the pleura. Approach should be transhepatic or transrenal only if necessary. Otherwise, the prone position (needle angled superiorly with the access caudal to the posterior sulcus) or lateral decubitus position (affected side down) may be used. For kidney masses, use US or CT from a lateral approach or prone posterior if needed. Retroperitoneal masses should be biopsied under CT guidance and rarely using ultrasound guidance. The posterior approach is suggested using large needles (19-gauge and up). If an anterior approach is indicated, be sure to avoid transgression of the bowel, or use a finer needle if absolutely necessary. For presacral and pelvic masses, CT guidance should be used. Splenic masses may be biopsied using CT or US guidance and should be performed with the intent to minimize the amount of parenchyma transgressed, due to the hypervascular nature of the organ and subsequent hemorrhage risk. Pancreatic masses are typically biopsied under endoscopic ultrasound, but sometimes lesions are amenable to fine needle aspiration percutaneously. Pancreatitis is the most obvious risk in these procedures, and can be avoided by careful avoidance of pancreatic parenchyma, including leaving out normal pancreatic tissue in the specimen provided. Biopsy of the liver parenchyma can be done via ultrasound guidance in most cases, with CT guidance necessary in some larger patients [36]. Organ-specific complications including bleeding risk estimates will be discussed ahead.

Postprocedure Management

Following the procedure, the patient should be kept under observation on bedrest for 2 h. When the patient's vital signs have stabilized and it has been confirmed that there have not been any complications resulting from the procedure, discharge is appropriate (expected 2–4 h). Immediately following procedure, a chest X-ray or CT taken on expiration is indicated to assess for development of pneumothoraces, in the case of lung biopsy and if pleural transgression may have occurred during the procedure. Heparin, LMWH, clopidogrel, aspirin, and NSAIDs can be reintroduced after 12 h postprocedure (low risk of bleeding) or 24 h post-risk procedure (high risk of bleeding). The patient should be aware of signs and symptoms of potential complications and be instructed properly on follow-up including provision of contact information.

Results

As the most common procedure performed by interventional radiologists, the technical success rate (diagnostic tissue retrieval) is expectedly high in percutaneous abdominal biopsy, estimated in 80–95% of cases [2]. Technical success is always increased with the demonstration of the needle tip within the lesion on imaging [24]. Sampling the necrotic portion of the lesion or an erroneous targeting of a smaller lesion decreases the viability of diagnosis.

Complications

Complications from percutaneous abdominal biopsy are rare, estimated at less than 2% [24, 37]. The most common (albeit, still rare with the greatest relative risk in renal biopsies) complication is hemorrhage which is usually controllable and depends on the organ implicated [24]: Hemorrhage in renal biopsy occurs in 0.5–6.6% of cases, especially when using larger needles (>18-gauge). Liver biopsies result in hemorrhage in an estimated 0.3–3.3% of cases, and splenic biopsies result in hemorrhage in up to 8.3% of cases. It is therefore important to consider the risk for hemorrhage in each patient prior to procedure, taking into account his or her coagulation status as well as the organ targeted for biopsy.

Infection is also very rare. In other rare instances, injury to adjacent viscera is possible. Pneumothorax is a risk and depends heavily on the route taken (impaction of the pleura). Needle tract tumor seeding is a rare scenario occurring in approximately 0.003–0.009% of cases. Mortality occurs in an estimated 0.006–0.031% of cases.

References

1. Wallace MJ, Chin KW, Fletcher TB, Bakal CW, Cardella JF, Grassi CJ, et al. Quality improvement guidelines for percutaneous drainage/aspiration of abscess and fluid collections. J Vasc Interv Radiol. 2010;21(4):431–5.
2. Kandarpa K, Machan L, Durham JD. Handbook of interventional radiologic procedures. 5th ed. Philadelphia: Wolters Kluwer; 2016. xxxiii, 613 p.
3. Valji K. Vascular and interventional radiology. 2nd ed. Philadelphia: Saunders Elsevier; 2006. xiii, 623 p.
4. Patel IJ, Davidson JC, Nikolic B, Salazar GM, Schwartzberg MS, Walker TG, et al. Consensus guidelines for periprocedural management of coagulation status and hemostasis risk in percutaneous image-guided interventions. J Vasc Interv Radiol. 2012;23(6):727–36.
5. McDermott VG, Schuster MG, Smith TP. Antibiotic prophylaxis in vascular and interventional radiology. AJR Am J Roentgenol. 1997;169(1):31–8.
6. Venkatesan AM, Kundu S, Sacks D, Wallace MJ, Wojak JC, Rose SC, et al. Practice guidelines for adult antibiotic prophylaxis during vascular and interventional radiology procedures. Written by the Standards of Practice Committee for the Society of Interventional Radiology and Endorsed by the Cardiovascular Interventional Radiological Society of Europe and Canadian Interventional Radiology Association [corrected]. J Vasc Interv Radiol. 2010;21(11):1611–30. quiz 31.
7. Sieber PR, Rommel FM, Agusta VE, Breslin JA, Huffnagle HW, Harpster LE. Antibiotic prophylaxis in ultrasound guided transrectal prostate biopsy. J Urol. 1997;157(6):2199–200.
8. Dravid VS, Gupta A, Zegel HG, Morales AV, Rabinowitz B, Freiman DB. Investigation of antibiotic prophylaxis usage for vascular and nonvascular interventional procedures. J Vasc Interv Radiol. 1998;9(3):401–6.
9. Health NCfCaI. NCCIH Clinical Research Toolbox.
10. Do H, Lambiase RE, Deyoe L, Cronan JJ, Dorfman GS. Percutaneous drainage of hepatic abscesses: comparison of results in abscesses with and without intrahepatic biliary communication. AJR Am J Roentgenol. 1991;157(6):1209–12.
11. Baijal SS, Agarwal DK, Roy S, Choudhuri G. Complex ruptured amebic liver abscesses: the role of percutaneous catheter drainage. Eur J Radiol. 1995;20(1):65–7.
12. Wronski M, Cebulski W, Slodkowski M, Krasnodebski IW. Minimally invasive treatment of infected pancreatic necrosis. Prz Gastroenterol. 2014;9(6):317–24.
13. Harisinghani MG, Gervais DA, Maher MM, Cho CH, Hahn PF, Varghese J, et al. Transgluteal approach for percutaneous drainage of deep pelvic abscesses: 154 cases. Radiology. 2003;228(3):701–5.
14. Maher MM, Gervais DA, Kalra MK, Lucey B, Sahani DV, Arellano R, et al. The inaccessible or undrainable abscess: how to drain it. Radiographics. 2004;24(3):717–35.
15. Beland MD, Gervais DA, Levis DA, Hahn PF, Arellano RS, Mueller PR. Complex abdominal and pelvic abscesses: efficacy of adjunctive tissue-type plasminogen activator for drainage. Radiology. 2008;247(2):567–73.
16. Gervais DA, Ho CH, O'Neill MJ, Arellano RS, Hahn PF, Mueller PR. Recurrent abdominal and pelvic abscesses: incidence, results of repeated percutaneous drainage, and underlying causes in 956 drainages. AJR Am J Roentgenol. 2004;182(2):463–6.
17. Zerem E, Imamovic G, Susic A, Haracic B. Step-up approach to infected necrotising pancreatitis: a 20-year experience of percutaneous drainage in a single centre. Dig Liver Dis. 2011;43(6):478–83.
18. Gotzinger P, Sautner T, Kriwanek S, Beckerhinn P, Barlan M, Armbruster C, et al. Surgical treatment for severe acute pancreatitis: extent and surgical control of necrosis determine outcome. World J Surg. 2002;26(4):474–8.

19. Rau B, Bothe A, Beger HG. Surgical treatment of necrotizing pancreatitis by necrosectomy and closed lavage: changing patient characteristics and outcome in a 19-year, single-center series. Surgery. 2005;138(1):28–39.
20. Akinci D, Akhan O, Ozmen M, Gumus B, Ozkan O, Karcaaltincaba M, et al. Long-term results of single-session percutaneous drainage and ethanol sclerotherapy in simple renal cysts. Eur J Radiol. 2005;54(2):298–302.
21. Rhodes A, Evans LE, Alhazzani W, Levy MM, Antonelli M, Ferrer R, et al. Surviving Sepsis Campaign: International Guidelines for Management of Sepsis and Septic Shock: 2016. Intensive Care Med. 2017;43(3):304–77.
22. Howell MD, Davis AM. Management of Sepsis and Septic Shock. JAMA. 2017;317(8):847–8.
23. Sainani NI, Arellano RS, Shyn PB, Gervais DA, Mueller PR, Silverman SG. The challenging image-guided abdominal mass biopsy: established and emerging techniques 'if you can see it, you can biopsy it'. Abdom Imaging. 2013;38(4):672–96.
24. Gupta S, Wallace MJ, Cardella JF, Kundu S, Miller DL, Rose SC, et al. Quality improvement guidelines for percutaneous needle biopsy. J Vasc Interv Radiol. 2010;21(7):969–75.
25. Lenders JW, Pacak K, Walther MM, Linehan WM, Mannelli M, Friberg P, et al. Biochemical diagnosis of pheochromocytoma: which test is best? JAMA. 2002;287(11):1427–34.
26. Tsou MH, Tsai SF, Chan KY, Horng CF, Lee MY, Chuang AY, et al. CT-guided needle biopsy: value of on-site cytopathologic evaluation of core specimen touch preparations. J Vasc Interv Radiol. 2009;20(1):71–6.
27. Chan D, Downing D, Keough CE, Saad WA, Annamalai G, d'Othee BJ, et al. Joint Practice Guideline for Sterile Technique during Vascular and Interventional Radiology Procedures: From the Society of Interventional Radiology, Association of periOperative Registered Nurses, and Association for Radiologic and Imaging Nursing, for the Society of Interventional Radiology [corrected] Standards of Practice Committee, and Endorsed by the Cardiovascular Interventional Radiological Society of Europe and the Canadian Interventional Radiology Association. J Vasc Interv Radiol. 2012;23(12):1603–12.
28. Sainani NI, Schlett CL, Hahn PF, Gervais DA, Mueller PR, Arellano RS. Computed tomography-guided percutaneous biopsy of isoattenuating focal liver lesions. Abdom Imaging. 2014;39(3):633–44.
29. Gupta S, Nguyen HL, Morello FA Jr, Ahrar K, Wallace MJ, Madoff DC, et al. Various approaches for CT-guided percutaneous biopsy of deep pelvic lesions: anatomic and technical considerations. Radiographics. 2004;24(1):175–89.
30. Tatli S, Gerbaudo VH, Feeley CM, Shyn PB, Tuncali K, Silverman SG. PET/CT-guided percutaneous biopsy of abdominal masses: initial experience. J Vasc Interv Radiol. 2011;22(4):507–14.
31. Krucker J, Xu S, Glossop N, Viswanathan A, Borgert J, Schulz H, et al. Electromagnetic tracking for thermal ablation and biopsy guidance: clinical evaluation of spatial accuracy. J Vasc Interv Radiol. 2007;18(9):1141–50.
32. Silverman SG, Gan YU, Mortele KJ, Tuncali K, Cibas ES. Renal masses in the adult patient: the role of percutaneous biopsy. Radiology. 2006;240(1):6–22.
33. Maturen KE, Nghiem HV, Caoili EM, Higgins EG, Wolf JS Jr, Wood DP Jr. Renal mass core biopsy: accuracy and impact on clinical management. AJR Am J Roentgenol. 2007;188(2):563–70.
34. Tam A, Krishnamurthy S, Pillsbury EP, Ensor JE, Gupta S, Murthy R, et al. Percutaneous image-guided splenic biopsy in the oncology patient: an audit of 156 consecutive cases. J Vasc Interv Radiol. 2008;19(1):80–7.
35. Li L, Liu LZ, Wu QL, Mo YX, Liu XW, Cui CY, et al. CT-guided core needle biopsy in the diagnosis of pancreatic diseases with an automated biopsy gun. J Vasc Interv Radiol. 2008;19(1):89–94.
36. Vijayaraghavan GR, David S, Bermudez-Allende M, Sarwat H. Imaging-guided parenchymal liver biopsy: how we do it. J Clin Imaging Sci. 2011;1:30.
37. Smith EH. Complications of percutaneous abdominal fine-needle biopsy. Review. Radiology. 1991;178(1):253–8.

Chapter 6
Biliary Interventions

Harry Griffin and Charan K. Singh

Percutaneous Cholecystostomy

Background

Percutaneous cholecystostomy is a procedure that involves the placement of a drainage catheter into the gallbladder to drain bile performed under image guidance [1]. The procedure is performed under local anesthesia, most commonly using ultrasound guidance. Commonly, the transhepatic approach is preferred due to reduced risk of biliary peritonitis or injury to the right colon. However, transperitoneal approach may be performed in coagulopathic patients at risk of bleeding from liver puncture.

Figure 6.1 illustrates the transhepatic approach to gaining access to the gallbladder using ultrasonography to visualize the relevant anatomy.

Indications

Percutaneous cholecystostomy is most commonly indicated for the management of acute cholecystitis, whether due to gallstones or otherwise [2].

In ICU patients with persistent sepsis and ultrasound demonstration of distended thick walled gallbladder with sludge, there should be a low threshold of placing a cholecystostomy tube. The contents of gallbladder can be cultured, and selective antibiotic regimen can be followed.

H. Griffin
University of Connecticut School of Medicine, Farmington, CT, USA

C. K. Singh (✉)
Department of Interventional Radiology, University of Connecticut Health Center, Farmington, CT, USA
e-mail: csingh@uchc.edu

© Springer International Publishing Switzerland 2018
C. K. Singh (ed.), *Gastrointestinal Interventional Radiology*, Clinical Gastroenterology, https://doi.org/10.1007/978-3-319-91316-2_6

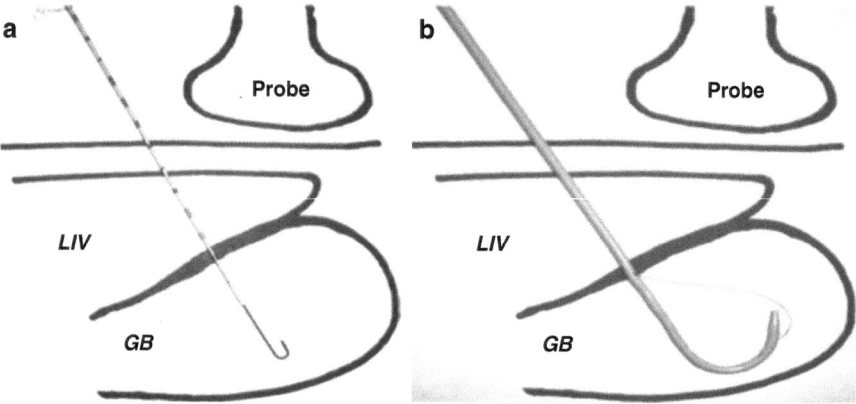

Fig. 6.1 (**a**) This figure demonstrates a transhepatic approach to gaining access to the gallbladder. The procedure is done under ultrasound guidance to guide needle entry into gallbladder lumen. A guidewire is then inserted as seen in this image. (**b**) Once access is established, the tract is dilated and a suture-activated locking pigtail catheter is placed, allowing for drainage

The second indication is gallstone cholecystitis in poor operative candidates. While laparoscopic cholecystectomy is the current standard of care, there is significant perioperative mortality in elderly and critically ill patients.

Contraindications

There are no absolute contraindications to percutaneous cholecystostomy. Relative contraindications include coagulopathy and contrast allergy (when performing under fluoroscopy). Coagulopathy can be reversed with a target platelet count above 50,000 per mL and international normalized ratio (INR) under 1.5.

Post-Procedural Care and Follow-Up

In immediate post-op, the patients should have bed rest, adequate analgesia, and continuance of antibiotics for at least 48 h. The drain should be flushed daily with 10 mL of sterile saline to prevent blockage.

Importantly, the drain needs to be left in place for at least 4–6 weeks to allow maturation of tract to the skin and prevent bile spillage into the peritoneum. A catheter check (Fig. 6.2) should be performed 4 weeks after the procedure to assess cystic and bile duct patency and can be removed, granted the cystic duct is patent and patient's clinical and blood test results are normal.

If stones are noted in CBD, ERCP would be indicated.

Fig. 6.2 Cholangiogram
performed 4 weeks after
percutaneous
cholecystostomy tube
placement demonstrating
patent cystic and common
bile duct with resolution of
cholecystitis. The patient's
clinical condition had
improved, and the catheter
can now be removed

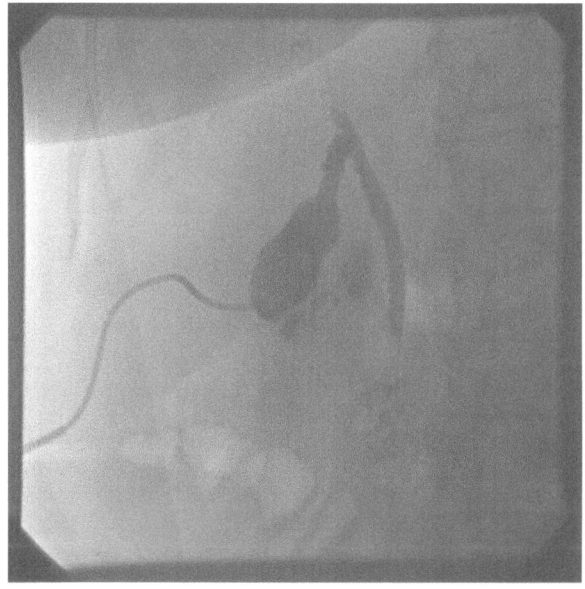

Outcomes and Complications

Percutaneous cholecystostomy has a high technical success rate. Often the tubes are placed bedside in the ICU patients with good outcomes and clearing of sepsis depending on patient's condition. Major complications include mortality, sepsis, and bleeding requiring transfusion. Mortality is very rare and is typically due to underlying patient comorbidities. Biliary infection is a risk of biliary instrumentation and can be mitigated with preoperative antibiotics.

Percutaneous Transhepatic Biliary Drainage

Background

Percutaneous transhepatic biliary drainage (PTBD) is an image-guided procedure that involves percutaneous access and drainage of the biliary tract. The procedure is performed in patients where endoscopic techniques are not possible or have failed in cases of surgically altered anatomy or a high biliary obstruction.

Frequently, an internal-external plastic catheter is placed that traverses the obstructive lesion with distal pigtail loop in the duodenum and proximal side holes above the obstruction (Fig. 6.3). In cases where there is failure to cross the tight obstruction, an external drain can be placed, and attempt at internalization can be performed in few days following biliary decompression.

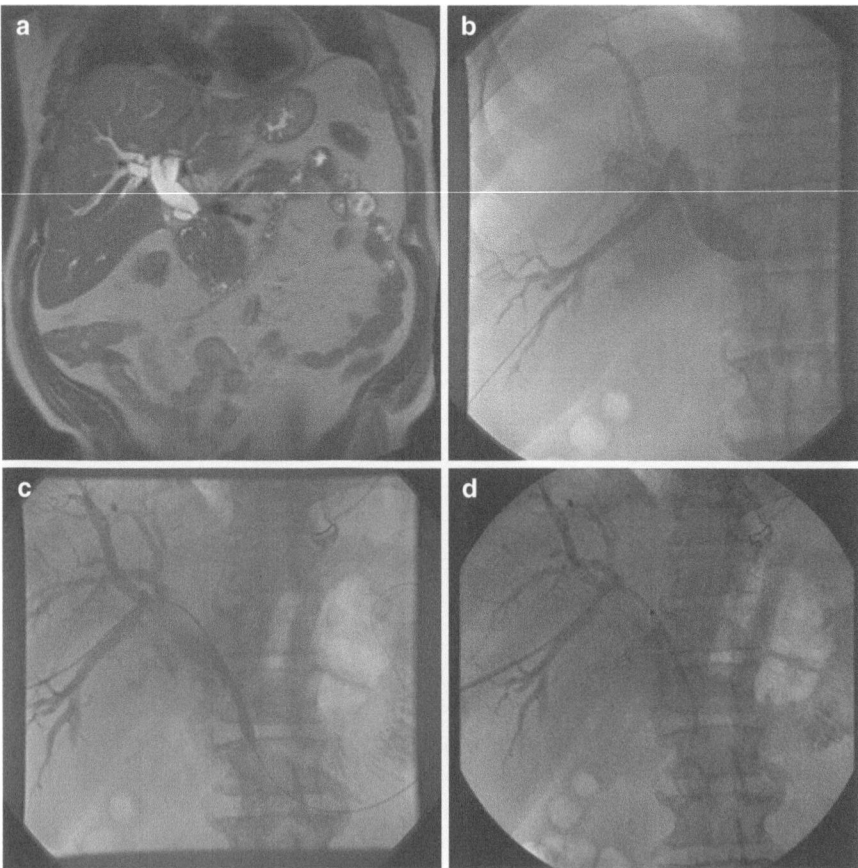

Fig. 6.3 (**a**) MRCP demonstrating dilated common bile duct and intrahepatic biliary obstruction. (**b**) Cholangiogram performed after gaining access to the right hepatic duct illustrating the level of the obstruction. (**c**) Successful passage of the guidewire past the obstruction and dilation of the obstructed common bile duct. (**d**) Placement of an internal-external plastic biliary drainage catheter across the previously obstructed common bile duct

Initially a drainage bag is attached to drain infected bile, and subsequently the bag is removed, and external catheter is capped to promote internal drainage, this way avoiding loss of biliary fluid and electrolytes. The catheter does require daily flushing to prevent occlusion and regular replacements (every 3 months or so).

Indications

Percutaneous transhepatic biliary drainage is safe and efficacious way to drain bile, which is often infected in patients with biliary obstruction.

The most common indications include the treatment of ascending cholangitis (urgent) and malignant biliary obstruction. Other indications include percutaneous treatment of choledocholithiasis, balloon dilatation of bilio-enteric anastomotic strictures. In cases of iatrogenic biliary fistula or leak, external drainage provides biliary diversion for fistula healing.

Contraindications

Contraindications to percutaneous transhepatic biliary drainage (PTBD) are relative and include coagulopathy and ascites. Intervention is generally considered safe with a platelet count above 50,000 per mL and an international normalized ratio (INR) under 1.5. Ascites can pose a technical challenge to PTBD; however patients with significant ascites can undergo paracentesis before biliary intervention.

Technique

The procedure is performed with the patient in the supine position. The skin area is cleaned and draped appropriately. Under ultrasound guidance, access into a peripheral biliary duct is gained. Once access is confirmed by backflow of bile, a guide wire is passed through the needle, which is then exchanged for a dilator. The guidewire is then removed, and a cholangiogram is performed to visualize the biliary duct anatomy and highlight the site of obstruction as seen in Fig. 6.3a. A catheter is then placed over the guidewire, which is advanced to the site of obstruction. Next, the guidewire is advanced past the obstruction into the duodenum. The site of the obstruction is then dilated using sequential dilators. Then, an internal-external drainage catheter is positioned across the narrowing and into the duodenum. The internal-external drainage catheter allows bile to drain externally into a collection bag or internally across the previously obstructed segment.

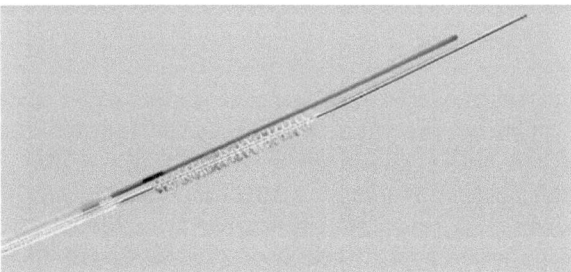

Endobiliary Tissue Sampling

Biliary cytology study can be performed on aspirated bile or with intraductal brush biopsy. Although these involve little risk, they are relatively insensitive (26–30%) in diagnosing biliary malignancy, particularly cholangiocarcinoma [5]. However, bile can be cultured in cases of acute cholangitis to guide appropriate antibiotics.

Post-Procedural Care and Follow-Up

Following transhepatic biliary drain placement, patients should have bed rest, adequate analgesia, and continuance of antibiotics for at least 48 h. The drain should be flushed daily with 10 mL of sterile saline to prevent blockage. The internal-external drain can be clamped after discussion with interventional radiology to promote internal drainage. The clamp should be removed and set to drain in cases of fever or new symptom onset.

Outcomes and Complications

With non-dilated biliary systems, the success of the procedure ranges from 60% to 96% [6]. Major complications include mortality, sepsis, and bleeding requiring transfusion. Mortality is very rare and is typically due to patient comorbidities. Biliary infection is an inherent risk of biliary instrumentation and can be mitigated with preoperative antibiotics. Post-procedural antibiotics can be considered on a case-by-case basis. Rarely, hemobilia due to arterial injury will require hepatic angiogram with coiling/occlusion of bleeding vessel.

Internal Biliary Stenting (Metal)

Background

Biliary duct stenting with internal bare metal stents is usually performed for palliative management of malignant biliary obstruction. It involves a metal stent that traverses the obstruction and allows bile to flow directly into bowel (Fig. 6.4) [3].

The stent is likely to remain patent for a longer period than most patient's life expectancy (median 6–8 months) [6, 7] and offers advantage of better lifestyle with no exiting catheter or need for catheter care. There is no external loss of biliary fluids or electrolytes. Disadvantage includes repeat PBD or endoscopic procedure in case of stent obstruction by tumor overgrowth [4].

Fig. 6.4 Coronal CT showing a successfully placed metal stent located in the distal common bile duct for palliation of inoperable malignant pancreatic mass

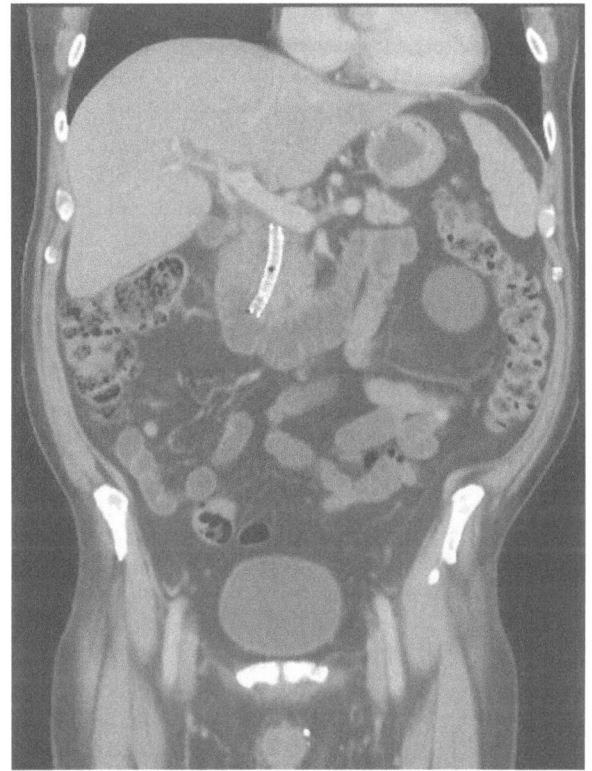

Indications

Biliary stents are commonly used to relieve obstruction caused by pancreatic malignancies, cholangiocarcinoma, or benign strictures following failed balloon angioplasty. Other indications include relieving obstruction caused by metastatic disease or external compression by lymphadenopathy.

Contraindications

There are no absolute contraindications for biliary stenting. Relative contraindications include coagulopathy, allergy to iodinated contrast agents, and ascites.

Pre-procedure Management

Patients with biliary obstruction should undergo contrast-enhanced computed tomography (CT) and/or magnetic resonance cholangiopancreatography (MRCP) to assess level of obstruction.

Figure 6.3a shows a MRCP in a patient with a known mass in the head of the pancreas with obstruction of distal CBD and dilation of the intrahepatic biliary system. MRCP provides a more detailed view of the biliary anatomy, extent of obstruction, and degree of dilation.

Laboratory testing should include assessment of the coagulation profile, including prothrombin time (PT) and international normalized ratio (INR). PT values should generally be within normal limits, and INR should be less than 1.5 for the procedure to be considered safe. Prophylactic antibiotics and intravenous fluids are typically given prior to starting the procedure.

Technique

Biliary stenting can be performed during the same percutaneous transhepatic biliary drainage procedure or afterward once the biliary system has been decompressed and an agreement with the surgical service regarding stent placement has been reached.

Access to the biliary system can be achieved using the same technique as described above with percutaneous transhepatic biliary drainage. Once access to the biliary tree is established, a cholangiogram should be performed to illustrate the site of obstruction and the relevant anatomy.

Once the site of the obstruction is traversed, a self-expanding metal stent can be placed. These stents can be covered or bare metal and expand when deployed. The bare metal stents are generally preferred due to their lower cost and low incidence of stent migration. However, they have a higher incidence of tumor ingrowth and blockage compared to covered stents. Figure 6.4 is a coronal CT demonstrating a successful placement of a metal stent in the distal common bile duct in a patient with a malignant obstruction.

Complications

The most common complications of biliary stent placement include occlusion and migration. Other complications include cholecystitis, pancreatitis, perforation, and bleeding. Stent occlusion and migration typically present with symptoms of abdominal pain and elevated liver enzymes indicative of cholestasis. Generally, computed tomography (CT) of the abdomen will be diagnostic for determining the etiology of the obstruction. Endoscopic retrograde cholangiopancreatography (ERCP) is frequently utilized for its ability to both diagnose and potentially treat obstructed stents.

Stent occlusion can occur due to tumor ingrowth into the stent, tumor growth causing compression of the stent, occlusion by biliary debris, or nonneoplastic tissue regeneration. The treatment requires placement of a plastic or metal stent within the original stent. Bleeding is a complication of biliary stent placement that can occur immediately after the procedure or later. Immediate postoperative bleeding can occur due to intrahepatic or extrahepatic bleeding from stent placement. Late bleeding can occur due to the formation of an arterial or venous biliary fistula.

Cholecystitis is a potential complication of biliary stent placement that is frequently seen when a covered stent is placed at or near the origin of the cystic duct. Pancreatitis is another potential complication of biliary stent placement secondary to manipulation of the distal bile duct, as is seen with ERCP.

References

1. Baron TH, Grimm IS, Swanstrom LL. Interventional approaches to gallbladder disease. N Engl J Med. 2015;373:357–65.
2. Horn T, Christensen SD, Kirkegård J, Larsen LP, Knudsen AR, Mortensen FV. Percutaneous cholecystostomy is an effective treatment option for acute calculous cholecystitis: a 10-year experience. HPB (Oxford). 2015;17:326–31.
3. Davids PH, Groen AK, Rauws EA, Tytgat GN, Huibregtse K. Randomised trial of self-expanding metal stents versus polyethylene stents for distal malignant biliary obstruction. Lancet. 1992;340:1488–92.
4. Li J, Li T, Sun P, Yu Q, Wang K, Chang W, Song Z, Zheng Q. Covered versus uncovered self-expandable metal stents for managing malignant distal biliary obstruction: a meta-analysis. PLoS One. 2016;11:e0149066.
5. Savader SJ, Prescott CA, Lund GB, et al. Intraductal biliary biopsy. Comparison of three techniques. J Vasc Interv Radiol. 1996;7:743.
6. Saad WEA, Wallace MJ, Wojak JC, Kundu S, Cardella JF. Quality improvement guidelines for PTC, biliary drainage and percutaneous cholecystotomy. J Vasc Interv Radiol. 2010;21:789.
7. Owens CA, Funaki BS, Ray CE Jr et al Expert panel on interventional radiology. ACR appropriate criteria. Radiologic management of benign and malignant biliary obstruction. 2008.

Chapter 7
Interventions in Portal Hypertension

Pushpinder Singh Khera

Portal hypertension is defined as an absolute portal venous pressure of greater than 10 mm Hg or the increase in portal venous-hepatic venous pressure gradient to more than 5 mm Hg [1].

Portal hypertension is one of the many manifestations of chronic liver disease. The three most common diseases leading to the latter are alcoholic liver disease, chronic viral hepatitis (hepatitis B and C virus related) and non-alcoholic steato-hepatitis (NASH).

The final common pathway in all cases of cirrhosis leading to portal hypertension is an increase in resistance to splanchnic blood flowing towards the liver. Therefore, the amount of blood flow in portal vein towards the liver decreases and it flows away from the liver into multiple porto-systemic collaterals in a bid to decrease the portal vein-hepatic vein pressure gradient. Figure 7.1 depicts the sequence of events that lead to development of portal hypertension in cirrhosis.

It is this alteration in portal blood flow haemodynamics that leads to the various complications of cirrhosis, namely ascites, haemorrhage from portosystemic varices (oesophageal, gastric or both), hepatic hydrothorax (refractory right-sided pleural effusion), hepatic encephalopathy and congestive splenomegaly. Figure 7.2 shows a schematic drawing of these complications.

The various interventions used to treat complications of portal hypertension are as follows:

P. Singh Khera
Department of Diagnostic and Interventional Radiology, All India Institute of Medical Sciences, Jodhpur, India
e-mail: kherap@aiimsjodhpur.edu.in

© Springer International Publishing Switzerland 2018
C. K. Singh (ed.), *Gastrointestinal Interventional Radiology*, Clinical Gastroenterology, https://doi.org/10.1007/978-3-319-91316-2_7

What happens in cirrhosis?

1. **Liver undergoes fibrosis (offers increased resistance to portal flow)**

2. **Increased hepatic vascular tone due to increased endothelin-1 production and decreased nitric oxide availability**

Increase in hepatic venous pressure gradient: HVPG> 10 mmHg

1. **Opening of porto-systemic collaterals leading to porto-systemic shunting and gastro-oesophageal varices formation**

2. **Ascites**

3. **Hepatic encephalopathy**

Fig. 7.1 Pathophysiology of cirrhosis leading to portal hypertension and its complications

TIPS (Trans Jugular Intrahepatic Portosystemic Shunt)

This procedure aims to decompress the portal circulation by creating a shunt through the hepatic parenchyma extending from one of the hepatic veins (usually the right hepatic vein but sometimes the middle hepatic vein) to the right branch of portal vein (Figs. 7.3 and 7.4). The procedure is done under general anaesthesia/deep sedation and involves accessing the jugular vein (mostly the right internal jugular) with subsequent extension of the hardware into the hepatic vein across the right atrium.

Indications for TIPS
Refractory ascites not responding to medical therapy such as paracentesis, diuretics, salt restriction: it responds very well to TIPS whereas paracentesis leads to protein and fluid loss every time it is done
Refractory hepatic hydrothorax (right-sided pleural effusion)
Acute/Recurrent variceal bleed not responding to endoscopic treatment
Budd Chiari syndrome (in this case the shunt extends from the IVC to the PV:Direct Intrahepatic Porto Caval Shunt)

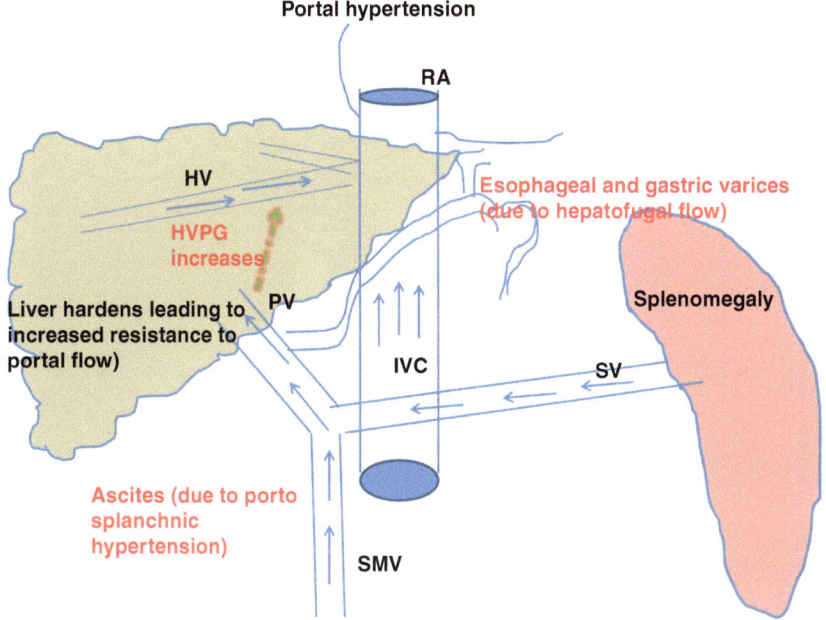

Fig. 7.2 Schematic diagram showing changes in haemodynamics occurring with development of portal hypertension and the consequent complications

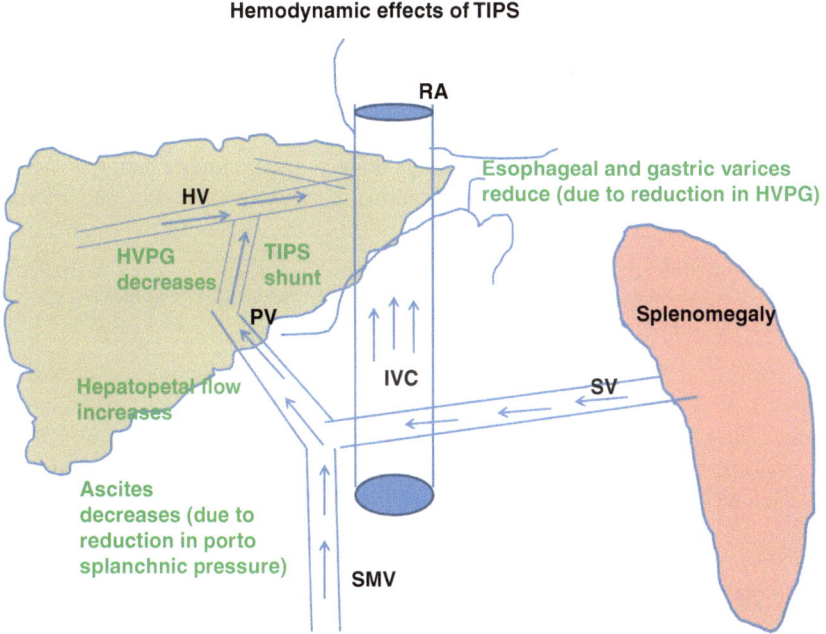

Fig. 7.3 Schematic diagram showing the haemodynamic changes occurring with creation of a TIPS shunt

Fig. 7.4 Image of a TIPS
procedure showing the
shunting of the blood
through the stent (red
arrow) extending from
right branch of portal vein
(yellow arrow) to the right
hepatic vein (green arrow)

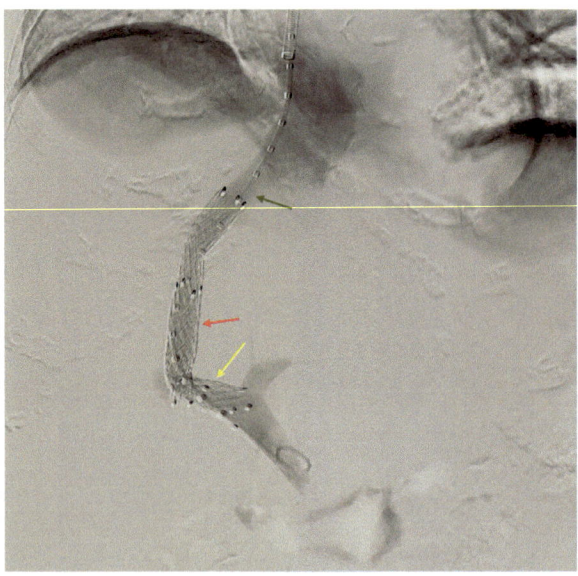

Contraindications for TIPS
Severe hepatic failure: MELD score of >18 is associated with a higher risk of early post TIPS mortality (this is so because TIPS per se leads to a decrease in portal flow to liver)
Severe heart failure: since there is increased volume load post TIPS
Severe biliary or systemic sepsis: post op infection rates are higher
Severe pulmonary hypertension: gets exacerbated post TIPS

Checklist Pre TIPS

- MELD score <18 (though TIPS can be done at a score higher than this value but the chances of post TIPS complications, e.g. encephalopathy and mortality, increase significantly) [2]
- Serum platelet count >60,000 per μL
- 2D Echo to rule out severe heart failure and pulmonary hypertension
- Rule out biliary/systemic infection

Ferral et al. [2] have mentioned a 30-day post TIPS mortality rate of 5–6% for patients with MELD score ≤17 undergoing elective TIPS for resistant ascites. The same figure for patients with MELD score ≥18 varied from 18 to 42%.

Mortality for patients undergoing emergency TIPS for non-responding bleeding oesophageal varices is more than in elective procedures for ascites [2].

Post TIPS Care and Follow-Up

- The patient should be in ICU/High dependency unit for the first 24 h post op with strict monitoring of vitals. Post TIPS ultrasound should be done at 48 h to ensure shunt patency

- Any serial increase in abdominal girth/abdominal pain should alert you to possibility of intra procedure capsular rupture: contact the operating interventional radiologist
- Early signs of hepatic encephalopathy and congestive heart failure must be recognized and corrective measures taken
- Liver functions tests should be sent at 24 h and 72 h and compared with baseline values to note any deterioration in liver function
- TIPS patient should attend the Interventional Radiology clinic at 6 weeks, 3 months and then at 6 monthly intervals for follow-up of TIPS shunt patency by Doppler evaluation

Post TIPS Complications

- Mild (8–10% of cases): access site haematoma, small pneumothorax, etc.
- Major (2–3% of cases): haemoperitoneum, sepsis, worsening of hepatic function, cardiopulmonary insufficiency (due to poor baseline cardiac reserve)
- Hepatic encephalopathy: may occur to a varying degree in up to 25–30% of cases post TIPS creation. Its incidence is maximum at 2–3 weeks post procedure. In most cases it responds favourably to medical management [3].

IVC Recanalization in Budd Chiari Syndrome

Obstruction of hepatic or suprahepatic IVC leads to congestion and eventually portal hypertension as a result of blockage of liver venous outflow.

The aetiology of IVC obstruction could be a membranous web in its supra hepatic segment. The same can be treated by angioplasty with large size balloons under conscious sedation with good long-term results.

If required the IVC can be stented too.

Hepatic Vein Recanalization in Budd Chiari Syndrome

Hepatic vein recanalization can be done for isolated hepatic venous outflow obstruction by means of angioplasty and stenting.

Key Points
- IVC and hepatic vein recanalization can delay or arrest the progression from a state of liver congestion to portal hypertension.
- Patients who undergo stenting of veins need to be on lifelong anticoagulation with maintenance of INR (International Normalized Ratio) between 2–2.5.
- They should undergo Doppler assessment at 3 months after the procedure and subsequently every 6 months to confirm stent patency.

Balloon Occluded Retrograde Transvenous Obliteration of Gastric Varices (BRTO)

BRTO is a procedure that aims to obliterate the large gastric varices in a case of portal hypertension which presents with either acute or chronic recurrent bleeding through a transvenous (femoral or jugular route) access. Such varices are difficult to control by endoscopic means. The connection between the gastric varices and left renal vein is a retroperitoneal vein: the gastrorenal shunt (GRS) and it is here that a balloon catheter is inflated so as to achieve stasis of sclerosant within the gastric varices and GRS (Figs. 7.5 and 7.6). The shunt and varices undergo thrombosis over a period of 6–8 h during which the balloon is kept inflated within the GRS. In addition to treat bleeding gastric varices BRTO is also useful to treat a patient of portal hypertension with large GRS on imaging who is having recurrent episodes of hepatic encephalopathy resistant to medical management.

Indications for BRTO
Acutely bleeding gastric varices
Large gastric varices at high risk of bleeding
Hepatic encephalopathy due to presence of a GRS which is not responding to medical therapy

The changes in haemodynamics after BRTO lead to an increase in hepatopetal (blood flow towards liver) and a theoretical risk in development of oesophageal varices and ascites. Hence these patients need to be on follow-up for the same.

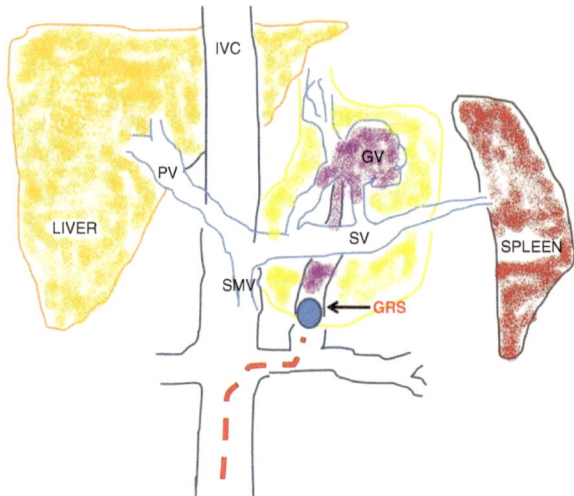

Fig. 7.5 Schematic diagram showing the placement of balloon catheter (dotted line) within the gastrorenal shunt (GRS) via the femoral route. The GRS and gastric varices show retention of sclerosant (violet colour) which eventually leads to thrombosis

Fig. 7.6 Image of a BRTO procedure done for a patient with child B stage chronic liver disease with recurrent bleeding from gastric varices. The black arrow highlights the occlusion balloon, the white arrow shows the gastrorenal shunt and the red arrow shows opacification of the gastric varices

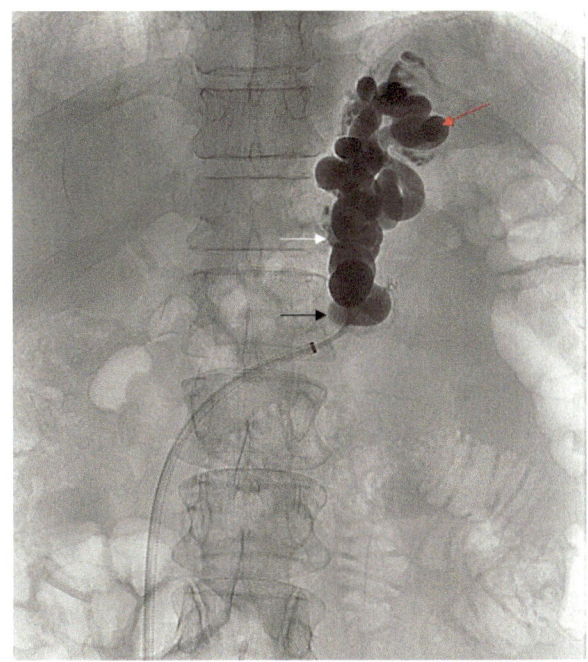

BRTO was previously done using ethanolamine oleate which had a risk of inducing haemolysis and haemoglobinuria. However nowadays it is done using sclerosant (sodium tetradecyl sulphate) which has a much better safety profile.

Transjugular Liver Biopsy (TJLB)

It is a safer alternative to percutaneous liver biopsy in patients with chronic liver disease under evaluation when coagulopathy and/or ascites preclude a percutaneous access. It has the advantage that hepatic venous pressure gradient can be done in the same sitting. It involves accessing the internal jugular vein and advancing an 18 G TruCut biopsy needle through a cannula under guidance into the hepatic parenchyma (Fig. 7.7).

Complications
- Liver capsular perforation
- Pseudoaneurysm formation
- Arteriovenous fistula formation

    Overall complication rate is <1%

Post Biopsy Care
- Watch vitals for 6 h
- Watch access site for hematoma

Fig. 7.7 Image of a TJLB
procedure showing the
biopsy needle (arrow)
advanced into the liver
through the right jugular
venous access

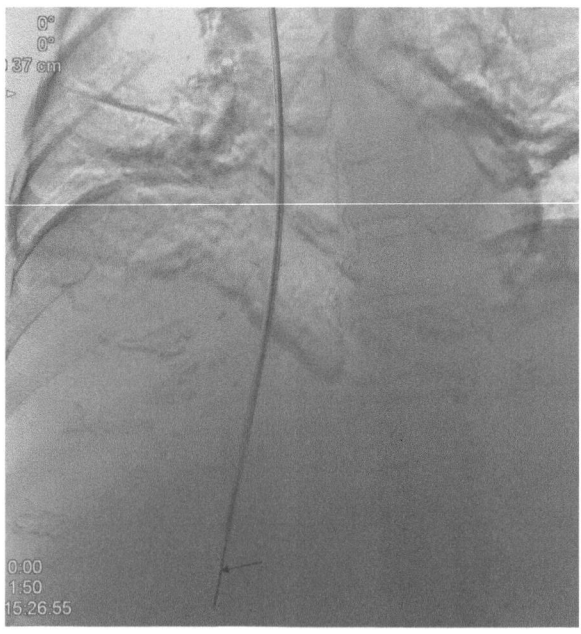

References

1. Merkel C, Montagnese S. Hepatic venous pressure gradient measurement in clinical hepatology. Dig Liver Dis. 2011;43:762–7.
2. Ferral H, Gamboa P, Postoak DW, Albernaz VS, Young CR, Speeg KV, McMahan CA. Survival
   after elective transjugular intrahepatic portosystemic shunt creation: prediction with model for
   end-stage liver disease score. Radiology. 2004;231:231–6.
3. Funes FR, Silva RCMA, Arroyo PC Jr, Duca WJ, Silva AAM, Silva RF. Mortality and complications in patients with portal hypertension who underwent transjugular intrahepatic portosystemic shunt (TIPS) – 12 years' experience. Arq Gastroenterol. 2012;49(2):143–9.

Suggested Reading

Kaufman JA, Bromley PJ. Portal and hepatic veins (chapter 14). In: Vascular and interventional
   radiology. 2nd edn. Elsevier Saunders; 2014.

Chapter 8
Liver: Oncology/Trauma

Elizabeth Anne C. Hevert and Suvranu Ganguli

Overview

Diseases of the liver are very common in both the pediatric and adult populations and often develop into chronic conditions. According to the Centers for Disease Control and Prevention (CDC), chronic liver disease and cirrhosis were the 12th leading causes of death in the United States [1]. Chronic hepatitis infection, alcoholic liver disease, and nonalcoholic fatty liver disease are by far the most common causes of chronic liver disease; however there are many other causes including genetic disorders, infections, toxins, autoimmune conditions, and trauma. As the incidence of chronic liver disease increases, so does the incidence of hepatocellular carcinoma (HCC), which has now become one of the most common causes of cancer-related deaths worldwide [2]. Interventional radiology plays a large role in the management of patients with liver disease including the treatment of ascites and portal hypertension and has a significant role to play in the management of hepatic tumors.

Many solid tissue malignancies including those involving the liver are poorly responsive to treatment regimens including systemic chemotherapy, surgical resection, and radiation therapy. Surgical resection, although fraught with high morbidity, remains the only potentially curative treatment for hepatic malignancies. However very few patients are suitable surgical candidates due to the prevalence of comorbid conditions. Minimally invasive image-guided therapies have thus become an appealing option and, with continued success, have become a widely accepted treatment strategy [3].

E. A. C. Hevert · S. Ganguli (✉)
Department of Interventional Radiology, Massachusetts General Hospital, Boston, MA, USA
e-mail: EHEVERT@mgh.harvard.edu; sganguli@mgh.harvard.edu

© Springer International Publishing Switzerland 2018
C. K. Singh (ed.), *Gastrointestinal Interventional Radiology*, Clinical
Gastroenterology, https://doi.org/10.1007/978-3-319-91316-2_8

HCC represents one the few cancers for which locoregional treatments can cure disease and prolong survival [4]. Although liver transplantation and resection remain the only treatment options with the potential for a cure, other treatment strategies may be employed to manage patients with advanced disease or can serve as a bridging therapy to transplant for patients with early or intermediate disease. Due to the complexity of treatment options, the decision for which treatment pathway to pursue should ideally be made by a multidisciplinary team that includes input from hepatology, oncology, interventional radiology, surgery, and pathology in order to ensure the best outcome for each patient. Several scoring systems have been developed in an attempt to categorize patients according to expected survival to help guide treatment decisions. The Barcelona Clinic Liver Cancer (BCLC) is the standard classification used for clinical management as it links the stage of disease with a recommended treatment strategy [5].

Hepatocellular Carcinoma

Overview

HCC is the fifth most common cause of cancer and patients with cirrhosis are at greatest risk for developing HCC [6]. The progression from a regenerative nodule to a dysplastic nodule and eventually a carcinoma is accompanied by the development of new arterial vessels that become the dominant blood supply to the tumor [7]. This feature is what allows HCC to be diagnosed by imaging alone, obviating the need for biopsy in many cases. The most typical finding is that of an arterially enhancing mass that demonstrates washout of contrast on delayed phase with the presence of a pseudocapsule of hyperenhancement on delayed phase imaging [8]. The characteristic arterial enhancement is because the tumor derives blood supply from abnormal hepatic arteries. The characteristic washout occurs during the portal venous phase when the normal liver parenchyma becomes hyper-attenuated, and the lesion is perceived as hypoattenuating in comparison [9]. The Liver Imaging Reporting and Data System (LIRADS) has standardized terminology and classified imaging findings for liver lesions and provides a score indicative of the relative risk for the described lesion to represent an HCC [10]. The Organ Procurement and Transplantation Network (OPTN) is also a standardized reporting system that classifies a lesion based on level of suspicion for malignancy and is used to determine patient eligibility and priority for transplantation [11]. When a nodule is larger than 1 cm in size in a cirrhotic patient and demonstrates arterial hyper vascularity with washout, the diagnosis of HCC can be made without the need for biopsy with a positive predictive value of 95% [12].

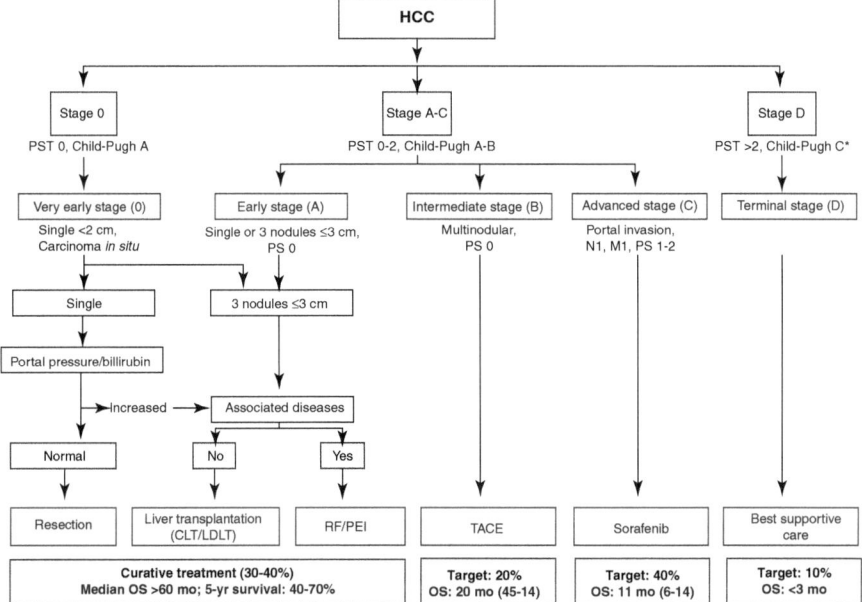

Fig. 8.1 The Barcelona Clinic Liver Cancer (BCLC) staging system and treatment strategy, 2011. *CLT* cadaveric liver transplantation, *LDLT* living donor liver transplantation, *OS* overall survival, *PEI* percutaneous ethanol injection, *RF* radio-frequency ablation, *TACE* trans-arterial chemoembolization

Staging and Treatment

Once the diagnosis of HCC has been made, the next step is in evaluating the potential options for treatment including surgical resection, transplantation, or percutaneous therapies. Owing to the fact that HCC typically occurs on a background of liver dysfunction and cirrhosis, tumor staging and treatment strategies depend not only on the size and spread of the tumor but also on the patients' underlying liver function and functional status [13]. The Barcelona Clinic Liver Cancer (BCLC) staging system takes into account the tumor stage and the patients' liver functional status, physical status, and cancer-related symptoms and classifies the patient as the following: very early stage, early stage, intermediate stage, advanced stage, and terminal stage (Fig. 8.1). The decision as to which treatment pathway to pursue should ideally be made by a multidisciplinary team using the BCLC staging system as a guide.

Very early-stage HCC is classified as the presence of a solitary small nodule, <2 cm in size, in a Child-Pugh A patient with no evidence of disseminated disease. In general, surgical resection is the treatment of choice for patients with very early-stage

HCC with preserved liver function and lack of portal hypertension. Percutaneous image-guided ablation can be offered as a first line therapy in patients who are not candidates for liver transplantation and is particularly useful when targets are not ideal for surgical excision [14].

Early-stage disease includes those patients with preserved liver function and a solitary HCC lesion or up to three nodules that are less than 3 cm in size. Surgical resection and liver transplantation are the best treatment strategies for these patients with studies demonstrating 60–80% 5-year survival [15]. Ablation techniques have been shown to be less efficacious when nodules are larger than 3 cm in size or when multinodular disease is present. Patients with tumors >5 cm in size are no longer considered transplant candidates, and these patients should be evaluated for possible surgical resection. The results of ablation in this population have been suboptimal, and patients should also be considered for trans-arterial chemoembolization (TACE) and radioembolization with ^{90}Y [16].

Patients classified as having intermediate-stage disease are those who have multinodular HCC with relatively preserved liver function with no evidence of vascular invasion or distant spread. These patients are generally referred for trans-arterial chemoembolization (TACE) or ^{90}Y radioembolization [17].

Advanced-stage HCC patients are those with vascular invasion or extrahepatic spread. These patients are typically treated with systemic therapy. There has been a lot of interest in the treatment of advanced-stage disease with radioembolization, particularly those with portal vein invasion; however the results are not decisive [18].

Liver transplantation remains the only option to provide a cure to the hepatoma as well as a cure to the underlying cirrhosis. Transplantation should be pursed in patients with an HCC smaller than 5 cm in size or three lesions each smaller than 3 cm in size with decompensated cirrhosis. Due to limited donor availability, oftentimes patients spend a considerable amount of time on the transplant wait list and frequently develop contraindications to transplantation within that time [19].

Tumor Ablation

Overview

Image-guided tumor ablation is a minimally invasive strategy to treat focal tumors by inducing cellular injury through the use of heat, cold, or chemicals and electrical current. The overall goal of focal tumor ablation is to completely treat the malignant cells within the target lesion as well as a rim of normal tissue that is presumed compromised due to microinvasion. Generally speaking, smaller lesions are more readily treated by percutaneous techniques; however larger tumors, defined as greater than 3–5 cm in diameter, can be treated using multiple ablation probes with overlapping ablation zones. Ablation procedures are typically performed under conscious sedation with standard cardiac, blood pressure, and oxygenation monitoring.

Chemical ablation is the image-guided instillation of a chemical agent such as ethanol or acetic acid that work by causing cellular dehydration, protein denaturation, and chemical occlusion of small vessels resulting in coagulative necrosis [20]. This type of ablation is most useful for treatment of encapsulated tumors such as HCC as the capsule prevents the ethanol from diffusing into normal hepatic parenchyma. The procedure is performed by the ultrasound-guided placement of a 19- to 21-gauge needle into the center of the tumor followed by instillation of absolute ethanol under direct sonographic visualization. The use of real-time imaging is helpful in order to monitor the volume of ethanol delivered and to ensure only a single tract is created from percutaneous entry site to the tumor to avoid spilling of ethanol into the peritoneal cavity. Chemical ablation with ethanol can result in complete necrosis in up to 70–80% of cases; however this technique requires multiple repeat interventions on a weekly basis until the desired volume is achieved [21]. The 5-year survival rate in patients with small tumors treated with chemical ablation range from 41–60% [22]. Chemical ablation is limited due to high local recurrence rates that are favored to be due to the inhomogeneous distribution of the chemical within the lesion.

Cryoablation is the process of causing tissue destruction and cell death by freezing. The tumor cells must be cooled to at least −35 °C degrees at which point mechanical destruction of the cell wall occurs resulting in cell death [23]. The process is achieved by the placement of cryoablation probes into the tumor, and this can be achieved by direct visualization in the setting of an open laparotomy or alternatively can be performed by the percutaneous image-guided placement of cryoprobes (see Fig. 8.2). CT guidance is the most preferred technique as once the "ice ball" forms, posterior acoustic shadowing occurs which limits visualization under ultrasound. Liquid forms of inert gases, typically argon gas or nitrogen, are cycled through the probes resulting in tissue cooling. Tissue necrosis occurs by the repetition of freeze and thaw cycles repeated two or three times per treatment. Freezing begins in the extracellular environment, thus water is drawn out from the cell resulting in osmotic dehydration. The high intracellular solute concentrations lead to protein damage and cell membrane injury [24]. The complication rates with hepatic cryoablation range from 15% to 50% and include the development of pleural effusions, hemorrhage, biliary fistula formation, abscess formation, and injury to adjacent organs or skin.

Hyperthermic ablation is performed through various techniques; however the goal is elevation of the cellular temperature above 50 °C degrees as this temperature induces denaturation of intracellular proteins and results in cell membrane destruction [23]. Thermal heat ablation techniques include the use of high-intensity focused ultrasound, also known as HIFU, microwave, and radio-frequency ablation (RFA).

High intensity focused ultrasound (HIFU) is performed by focusing of multiple small piezoelectric crystals to deposit energy in the form of sound to induce heat destruction [25]. The benefit of HIFU is that the focused energy is transmitted transcutaneously into the target, therefore obviating the need for percutaneous probe placement. The drawback to HIFU is that it is time-consuming since the focused beam is very small, thus requiring longer ablation times.

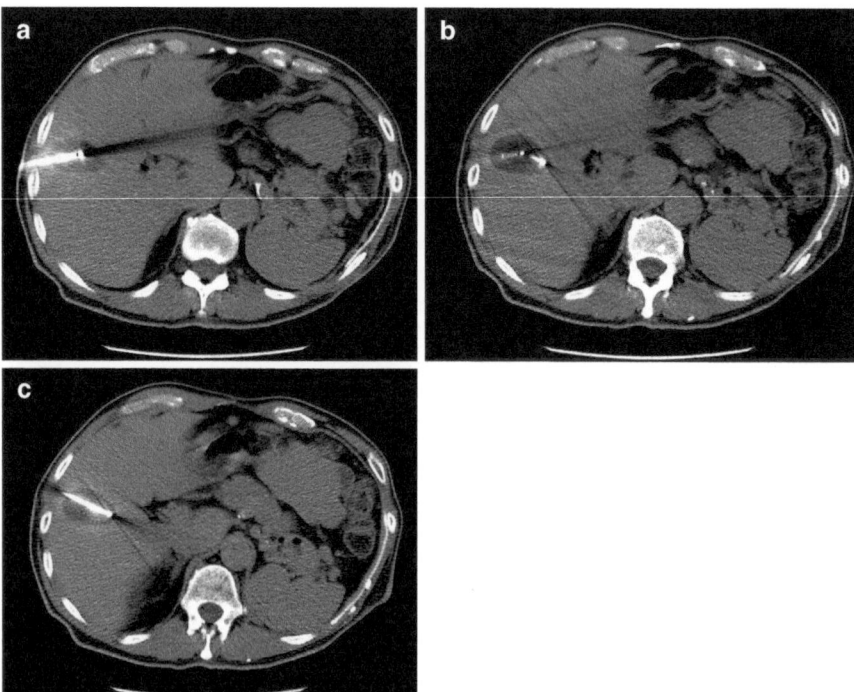

Fig. 8.2 Image-guided cryoablation. (**a–c**) Axial images through the tumor demonstrating probe positioning. Two separate 17-gauge cryoablation probes are demonstrated placed percutaneously under CT guidance into the right lobe liver tumor. Easy visualization of the ice ball facilitates monitoring the ablation zone to avoid injury to adjacent structure

RFA is by far the most well-studied ablation technique. During RFA, energy is created by alternating electrical currents resulting in agitation of ions and frictional heat that subsequently results in coagulation necrosis. RF ablation is a safe, predictable, and effective means to treat solid neoplasms via percutaneous approach. As with cryoablation, the RF probe is inserted into the tumor using image guidance and the RF probe creates and electrical circuit within the patient between an active probe within the tumor and large dispersive grounding pads placed on the patient's thigh or back. RF ablation is limited due to the inverse relationship between heat depositions with increased distance from the energy source; therefore, the tissue temperature rapidly declines at increasing distance from the probe [26]. Additionally, RF is limited in the presence of large blood vessels since flowing blood results in dissipation of heat, also known as the "heat sink" effect. As with cryoablation, RF ablation can be performed in the open operative setting; however percutaneous RF probe placement has the advantage of being a minimally invasive technique that can be performed under conscious sedation as opposed to subjecting the patient to general

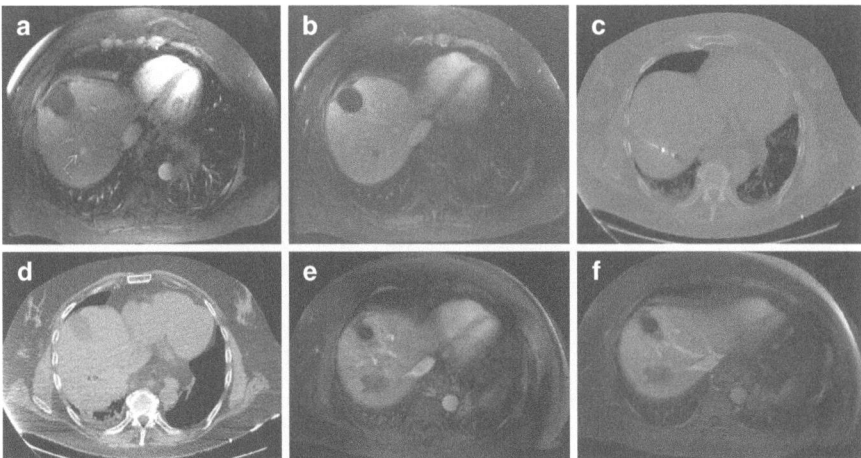

Fig. 8.3 Image-guided microwave ablation. (**a**) Axial contrast-enhanced MRI in the arterial phase demonstrates the enhancing liver lesion. (**b**) Axial contrast-enhanced MRI in the delayed venous phase demonstrates washout of the liver lesion. (**c**) Axial CT image during microwave ablation demonstrates the single 14-gauge microwave probe placed percutaneously under CT guidance into the right lobe liver tumor. (**d**) Axial CT image after microwave probe removal demonstrates small foci of gas within the treated segment of the liver, an expected posttreatment finding. (**e**) Axial contrast-enhanced MRI in the arterial phase performed 4 weeks after treatment demonstrates resolution of the previously noted arterial enhancement. (**f**) Axial contrast-enhanced MRI in the delayed venous phase performed 4 weeks after treatment demonstrates large area of hypointensity consistent with tumor necrosis

anesthesia. The standard RF ablation probes are between 17- and 14-gauge in outer diameter, which translates to between 1.15 and 1.63 mm. RF ablations of HCC are associated with very low mortality rates ranging from 0.1% to 0.5% and are most commonly from sepsis, hepatic failure, colonic perforation, or portal vein thrombosis. Common major complications include intraperitoneal bleeding, hepatic abscess formation, bile duct injury, and hepatic decompensation occurring in approximately 2.2–3.1% of patients [27].

Microwave ablation utilizes a thin, 14-gauge, antennae inserted into the target tissue through which energy is applied (see Fig. 8.3). The microwave generator emits an electromagnetic wave, and the energy applied to the tissues results in rotation of polar water molecules. Frictional forces oppose that induced rotation and the rotational energy is converted to heat [28]. The rotation generated results in a uniform distribution of heat, the shape and size of which can be altered based on the type of needle selected. The potential benefits of microwave technology over RF ablation include higher intra-tumoral temperatures with larger tumor ablation zones and faster ablation times [29].

Irreversible electroporation is technically a nonthermal ablative technique, whereby the cells are exposed to repeating pulses of an electrical current, which

Fig. 8.4 Image-guided
irreversible electroporation

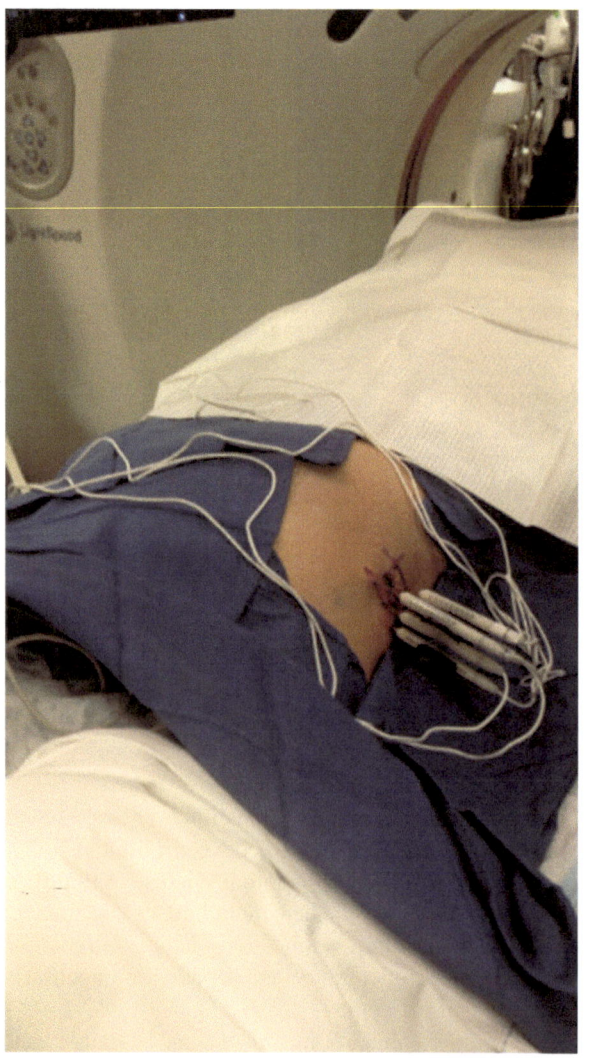

generates an electrical field that irreversibly damages the cell membrane leading to apoptosis [30]. The benefit of IRE is that this technique is less damaging to surrounding tissues such as collagenous tissues and nerves. The downside to IRE is that most treatments require multiple probes spaced 1–3 cm apart in order to create the electrical field strong enough to induce irreversible cell death (see Fig. 8.4). Additionally, IRE is limited as it must be performed under general anesthesia with muscle blockade due to the potential to induce cardiac arrhythmias and muscle contractions.

Patient Selection for Ablation

Various imaging modalities are commonly employed in determining the diagnosis of a patient who presents to the hospital or clinic with a complaint. Very often, lesions are incidentally found in the liver on an ultrasound or CT scan that are performed for abdominal pain. Liver masses are also discovered in those patients who receive imaging for routine surveillance in the setting of a known malignancy or cirrhosis. If a mass is discovered, frequently a second diagnostic imaging modality is recommended in order to properly evaluate the lesion. Proper technical evaluation of a mass should be performed with the use of a contrast-enhanced CT or MRI. As previously discussed, many times imaging features are sufficient to characterize a mass lesion as malignant; however in those cases when imaging findings are inconclusive, a biopsy should be performed.

Once a lesion has been deemed a malignancy by either imaging or a positive biopsy, evaluation of the patient's clinical status as well as potential ability to undergo treatment should be performed, and often this should be accomplished through a multidisciplinary meeting. Those tumors that can be safely resected for a cure should undergo a surgical evaluation. A good working relationship with persons from the multidisciplinary team including medical oncology, surgical oncology radiation oncology, and interventional oncology is essential in the treatment of these patients. Relative contraindications to thermal ablation include the presence of excessive tumor burden, diffuse or distant metastatic disease, and an active infection or uncorrectable severe coagulopathy. Additionally, evaluation of relevant imaging in order to determine a safe and effective pathway for placement of the ablation probes should be performed. A careful evaluation of adjacent structures that can potentially make ablation less efficacious should be performed such as evaluation for large portal or hepatic veins due to "heat sink" and for the presence of structures that have the potential for clinically significant injury following ablation such as the diaphragm, gallbladder, or large bile ducts.

Whether performing cryoablation, microwave ablation, or RF ablation, the procedure is performed via the percutaneous placement of ablation probes; therefore investigation of patients' coagulation profile and platelet function should be performed before the procedure. Additionally, the use of anticoagulants including antiplatelet agents should be stopped a sufficient time before the procedure. An up-to-date knowledge of existing anticoagulants and timing interval for holding these medications is crucial prior to scheduling a patient for this type of procedure. Often it is necessary to consult the ordering physician to ensure if it is safe to hold these medications. Additional pre-procedure laboratory studies should be obtained including a complete blood count to evaluate for infection or severe anemia and thrombocytopenia; blood chemistries including AST, ALT, alkaline phosphatase, and bilirubin; and appropriate tumor markers such as AFP if applicable. A baseline EKG should be performed and as a precaution, one should obtain a blood type and cross match.

On the day of the procedure, the operator should familiarize themselves with the imaging and prepare a strategy for pre-procedure pain management, patient positioning for probe placement, and the possibility of post-procedure admission either related to uncontrolled pain or procedure-related complication.

Ablation Procedure and Post Procedure

Ablation can be performed with the patient under conscious sedation achieved with intravenous administration of midazolam and fentanyl, for example. Certain circumstances including the presence of multiple medical comorbidities may require anesthesia consultation. Patients undergo monitoring with continuous pulse oximetry and electrocardiography. Vital signs including heart rate, blood pressure, and oxygen saturation should be monitored every 5 min.

A post-procedure treatment protocol should be established in order to closely monitor patients for pain and/or complications. Typically, patients require an overnight stay in the hospital with a generous pain medication regimen, oftentimes through the use of a PCA pump. The patient must be successfully transitioned from IV medication to oral medications and should be ambulatory and tolerating a diet before discharge. The patient should return to the clinic for a follow-up approximately 4 weeks from the procedure and should receive imaging either with a contrast-enhanced MRI or CT. Imaging earlier than 4 weeks often leads to false negative findings of residual disease due to the presence of posttreatment inflammation. If the patients are found to have residual disease on the follow-up imaging, patients can be considered for repeat treatment.

Chemoembolization

Overview

Arterial embolization techniques are the primary therapy for the treatment of HCC in more advanced stages in patients who are not surgical candidates. The goal of chemoembolization is to combine the effects of local ischemia with the delivery of a high local concentration of chemotherapeutic medications [31]. As previously discussed, HCC lesions derive their blood supply from the hepatic arterial system in contrast to the normal liver parenchyma that derives a majority of blood flow from the portal system. This altered blood flow distribution is what is exploited in the treatment of HCC with embolic therapy be it chemoembolization, radioembolization, or bland particle embolization.

Hepatic arterial embolization can be performed with the use of microembolic particles that are delivered into the tumor arterial supply and are small enough to reach and interrupt the blood supply to the tumor at the capillary level. Selective embolization of hepatic arterial supply to tumors results in tumor ischemia with relative sparing of the normal hepatic parenchyma. In chemoembolization, ethiodized oil mixed with chemotherapy followed by microspheres or microsphere particles formulated to absorb chemotherapeutic drugs is delivered via the arterial blood supply directly to the target tumor. These treatments occlude the small arterial branches, causing tumor ischemia, and result in high concentrations of chemotherapy in the tumor microenvironment [32]. If the particles are used alone for embolization, this is termed bland embolization. The theoretic advantage for TACE is the ability to deliver high concentrations of potent drugs to a local environment that has become more sensitized to the effects of chemotherapy under conditions of ischemia [33]. There is some controversy regarding the topic of bland embolization versus chemoembolization; however, there are no randomized control trials that have demonstrated a clear advantage of adding chemotherapy to the particles [34, 35].

Patient Selection

Chemoembolization should be used in the treatment of unresectable HCC in patients with relatively preserved liver function. Additionally, chemoembolization has a role in the treatment of patients who are on the wait list for liver transplant in order to prevent disease progression that may preclude them from receiving a transplant [36]. Patients with decompensated liver failure or at high risk for liver failure should not undergo chemoembolization nor should those patients with poor performance status as they are not likely to benefit from this line of therapy.

Procedure

The procedure can be performed with intravenous conscious sedation using a combination of Fentanyl and Versed. A detailed review of relevant pre-procedure imaging is necessarily to evaluate the levels at which the visceral vessels originate, the distribution and take off of the arterial supply to the tumor and to evaluate for anatomic variants. In order to perform catheter-directed therapies safely and effectively, the operator must be very familiar with the hepatic arterial anatomy and common variations (see Fig. 8.5). A replaced hepatic artery is a normal anatomic variant in which the right hepatic artery arises from the superior mesenteric artery as opposed to the celiac axis (see Fig. 8.6). Commonly, an accessory hepatic artery is identified in pre-procedure imaging or at the time of angiography, and in these cases, both a right hepatic artery arising from the proper hepatic artery is seen as well as a hepatic arterial branch arising from the SMA. In addition to a careful angiographic evaluation of the celiac and superior mesenteric arteries, the phrenic branches should be interrogated as they are frequently recruited by the tumor vasculature.

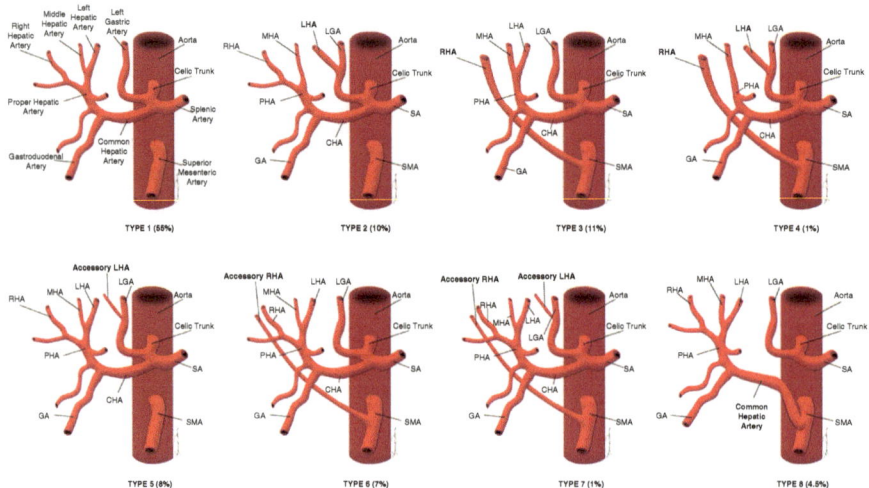

Fig. 8.5 Classification of hepatic arterial anatomy. Used with permission from Massachusetts General Hospital

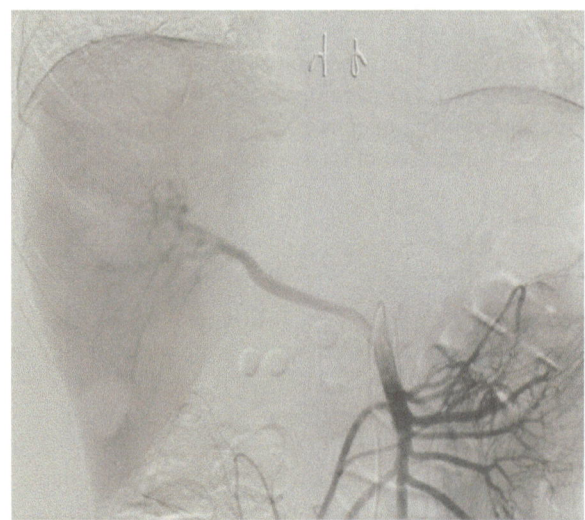

Fig. 8.6 Replaced hepatic artery. DSA from the superior mesenteric artery demonstrates the presence of a replaced hepatic artery supplying the right lobe of the liver

Pre-procedure prophylactic antibiotics are routinely suggested and are particularly important in those patients with biliary stenting as those patients are at increased risk for hepatic abscess formation. Arterial access is obtained either through the common femoral artery or the left radial artery using a micropuncture system that is exchanged over a 0.035″ wire for a 5F vascular sheath. Typically, a 4F or 5F catheter is used to select the visceral arteries, and digital subtraction angiograms (DSA) are performed of both the celiac axis and the superior mesenteric

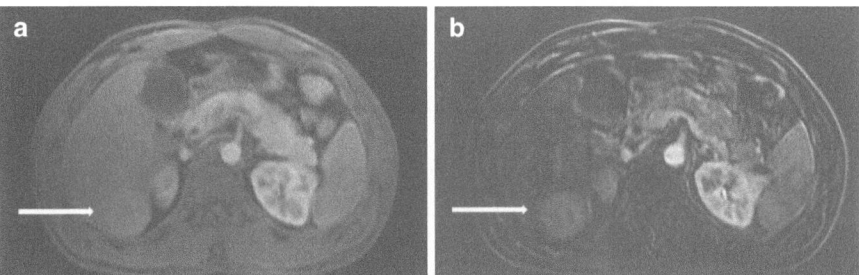

Fig. 8.7 Patient referred for TACE pre-procedure MRI. (**a**) Axial contrast-enhanced MRI of the abdomen during the arterial phase. White arrow denotes enhancing mass in the posterior right hepatic lobe. (**b**) Axial contrast-enhanced MRI of the abdomen on subtracted arterial phase. White arrow again denotes the enhancement of the mass on the subtracted arterial phase sequence

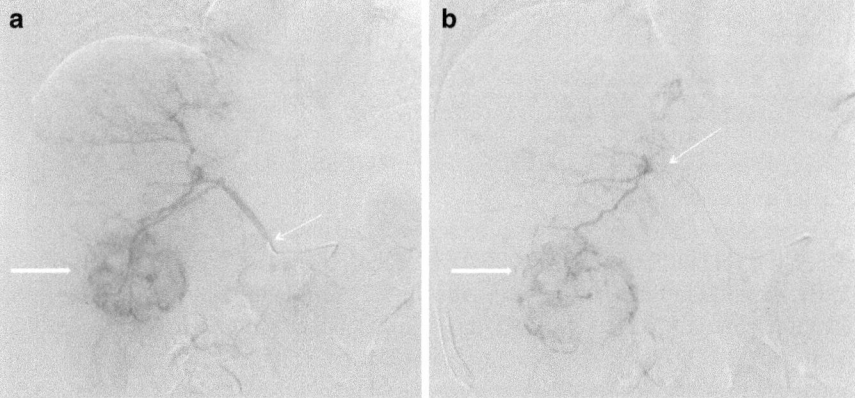

Fig. 8.8 Patient referred for TACE intra-procedure imaging. (**a**) DSA of the liver. The 5Fr catheter tip is within the proper hepatic artery, denoted by the skinny white arrow. The thick white arrow denotes the tumor blush. (**b**) A 2.8Fr micro-catheter, denoted by the skinny white arrow, has been advanced into the segmental branch supplying the tumor. The tumor blush is again seen, as denoted by the thick white arrow

artery to further elucidate the arterial supply of the tumor (see Fig. 8.7). The arteriogram should be carried out until the portal vein is visualized to document adequate portal flow. A careful review of the arteriogram should be performed to confidently identify the gastric arteries and gastroduodenal artery to avoid nontarget embolization that may result in bowel or stomach infarction. If there is any doubt regarding the arterial supply to the tumor, a cone-beam CT scan can be performed to identify feeding vessels. A 2.8 French or 3.0 French micro-catheter and 0.018″ micro-wire combination are subsequently used to select the appropriate hepatic artery and to navigate the arterial supply of the tumor using the DSA as a roadmap for catheter positioning. Proper positioning of the micro-catheter for the delivery of embolic particles is crucial since proximal arterial occlusion stimulates collateral vascular supply to the tumor, and treatments are not effective (see Fig. 8.8). In addition,

Fig. 8.9 Patient referred for TACE intra-procedure imaging. DSA of the liver following delivery of microembolic agents. The thick white arrow is at the site of previously seen tumor blush. The tumor blush is no longer visualized consistent with successful treatment

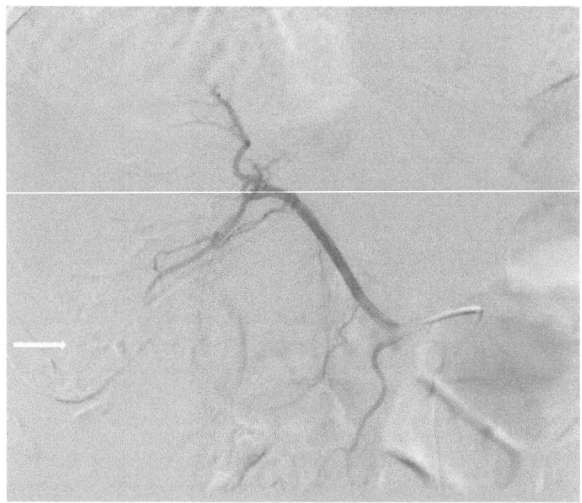

permanent arterial occlusion to the tumor segments with coils, for instance, is not desirable as this precludes repeat intervention if needed in the setting of collateral vessel formation.

Once satisfactory catheter positioning has been obtained as confirmed by a repeat DSA, the chemotherapy agents can be delivered. The embolization agents are typically 100–300 μm particles mixed with contrast, and in the setting of chemoembolization, commonly used chemotherapeutic agents include doxorubicin, epirubicin, and cisplatin. The microembolic agents are injected under real-time fluoroscopic guidance to watch for reflux of contrast into nontarget vessels suggesting the force of injection is too great. Additionally, the injection is performed under fluoroscopic guidance to look for slowing and eventual stasis of contrast within the targeted vascular supply. After embolization is complete, a post-embolization angiogram is typically performed using a hand-injected DSA from the micro-catheter often followed by a power-injected DSA from the 4 or 5 French catheter (see Fig. 8.9). A careful review of these post-embolization angiograms should be performed as they may show the presence of a prominent feeding vessel to the tumor that was masked on the initial angiogram by the presence of the now embolized vasculature.

Post Procedure

As with patients who are treated with ablation, patients are often admitted overnight after embolization to monitor for complication and to treat post-procedure pain. Post-embolization syndrome occurs in 60–90% of patients and manifests with pain, fever, nausea, and vomiting and can last for several hours to a few days. Patients can be discharged to home once they are tolerating a diet, are ambulatory, and have

Fig. 8.10 Patient referred for TACE post-procedure follow-up imaging. Axial contrast-enhanced MRI of the abdomen in the arterial phase denotes an interval resolution of the previously seen enhancement within the tumor located in the posterior aspect of the right lobe, denoted by the thick white arrow

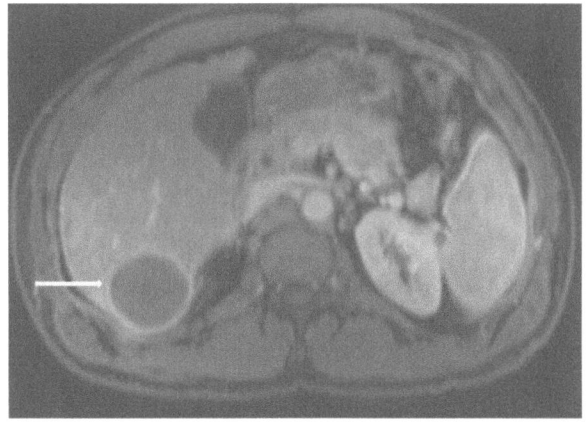

transitioned to parenteral narcotics. As with post-ablation patients, the patients should return to clinic in 4 weeks with a follow-up contrast-enhanced CT or MRI (see Fig. 8.10). Major complications include the development of hepatic insufficiency, hepatic abscess formation, and nontarget embolization. Studies have demonstrated a benefit of chemoembolization on patient survival. In comparing chemoembolization versus conservative management, a 2-year survival benefit has been shown with chemoembolization; however patient selection is key [37]. Patients who undergo chemoembolization with decompensated liver function or poor functional status do not demonstrate the same survival benefit.

Radioembolization

Overview

Radioembolization is a catheter-based delivery of microparticles that serves to occlude the small vessels supplying the tumor resulting in ischemia combined with the local delivery of radiation therapy with Yttrium 90. The benefit of such therapies is in the ability to limit radiation exposure to the liver and reduce the risk of radiation-induced liver disease (RILD) [38]. Radioembolization is used for the treatment of unresectable liver cancer including metastatic disease and primary HCC. There are two types of microspheres available that both contain Yitrium (^{90}Y) as the active particle but have different carriers: ^{90}Y glass microspheres called TheraSpheres and ^{90}Y glass resin-based microspheres called SIR-spheres [39]. ^{90}Y is a pure beta emitter with emitted electrons having an average tissue penetration depth of approximately 2.5 mm. ^{90}Y microspheres once injected in the arterial supply of a tumor will emit radiation that will penetrate the tissue a maximum of 10 mm from the injection site; therefore the patient being treated poses no threat to others [40]. The half-life of ^{90}Y is 64.2 h, so the majority of the radiation emitted after treatment ceases after 10–14 days.

Patient Selection

As was discussed with chemoembolization, in an ideal scenario a multidisciplinary panel meets to review patient eligibility for treatment. Included in this evaluation are the patient's clinical history, pertinent physical exam findings, and laboratory evaluation including liver and renal function assessment. The selection criteria are similar to those patients who are treated with TACE. Cross-sectional imaging preferably with a contrast-enhanced MRI of the abdomen should be performed to calculate tumor volume and evaluate anatomy prior to treatment. Due to the risk of nontarget embolization with ^{90}Y therapy, a pretreatment planning visceral angiogram must be performed to delineate vascular anatomy, provide the operator an opportunity to prophylactically coil vascular territories at risk for nontarget embolization, and detect extrahepatic shunting. Celiac and superior mesenteric artery diagnostic visceral angiograms are performed as well as sub-selective hepatic arteriograms to map out the vascular anatomy of the tumor and define collateral vessels or variant anatomy that may require prophylactic embolization. Prophylactic embolization of the gastroduodenal artery or the right gastric artery may be necessary in select populations as this procedure is generally of no clinical consequence owing to the profound vascular collaterals; however nontarget embolization with ^{90}Y in these areas can lead to significant morbidity [41]. HCC tumors commonly are associated with arteriovenous intra-tumoral shunting; therefore, pretreatment assessment of the shunt fraction must be determined in order to avoid excess radiation to the lungs and possible radiation pneumonitis. The assessment of lung shunt fraction is performed after the diagnostic angiograms for vascular mapping have been performed, and the location for treatment has been precisely determined. After which, the micro-catheter is placed at the location of intended treatment; however instead of delivering the ^{90}Y, technetium-labeled albumin (^{99}Tc-MAA) is delivered. The patient is subsequently transported to the nuclear imaging department where the ratio of delivered ^{99}Tc-MAA dose relative to the dose noted in the lungs is calculated. A shunt fraction greater than 10% if using glass microspheres or greater than 20% if using resin-based microspheres generally precludes the patient from receiving radioembolization with ^{90}Y [42].

Procedure

The technique for the delivery of intra-arterial ^{90}Y radioembolization is similar to that of chemoembolization. The information obtained from the pretreatment angiogram is reviewed as the vascular anatomy has been previously mapped and the location of treatment has already been determined. Common femoral artery access is obtained typically using a micropuncture set with upsize to a 0.035″ wire and 5F vascular sheath. A 5F Cobra or 5F Simmons-1 catheter can be used to select the celiac or superior mesenteric artery, depending on what was determined in the pretreatment evaluation, followed by the placement of a micro-wire and 3F micro-catheter. Once the micro-catheter is properly positioned, the ^{90}Y microspheres can be delivered to the desired target treatment area. The delivery of the microspheres must be performed with adequate pressure so as to avoid the ^{90}Y particles from falling out of suspension; however care must be taken to avoid applying too much pressure that may result in reflux of adjacent proximal vessels resulting in unintended nontarget embolization. Care must be taken with delivering the ^{90}Y embospheres, and proper radiation handling and disposal should be performed according to institutional standards.

Post Procedure

Most patients are discharged the same day. Postoperative evaluation should include evaluation for common procedure adverse effects include arterial puncture complications, edema, GI symptoms including gastritis, and hepatic decompensation. Patients should be informed of possible treatment-related side effects including the possibility of post-radioembolization syndrome that can occur within 1 to 2 days posttreatment presenting as fatigue, nausea, vomiting, fever, and abdominal pain. Post-procedure laboratory derangements are common including elevation in serum bilirubin and transient elevation in transaminases; however these findings should return to pretreatment baseline within 2–3 weeks. Patients should return to the clinic for follow-up evaluation with imaging approximately 4–6 weeks after treatment. The most important factors evaluated in determining the need and eligibility of a patient for further treatment is the tumor response as seen on cross-sectional imaging, the patient's pre- and posttreatment performance status, and the patient's liver function.

Clinical Outcomes

Severe complications including liver toxicity, pneumonitis, gastrointestinal bleeding or ulceration, and death have been reported. The risk factors that have been established associated with morbidity and mortality are related to available liver reserve with those patients with low reserve are at increased risk for adverse events [43]. Radiation-induced liver disease has an incidence rate of 0–4% and occurs between 4 and 8 weeks from treatment and is associated with radiation doses of 150Gy. Long-term sequela of treatment can include liver fibrosis that can result in portal hypertension; however, this is more commonly seen in those patients with bi-lobar treatment or in patients with preexisting cirrhosis.

Radioembolization is a therapeutic option for patients with intermediate-stage HCC and has shown to demonstrate longer time to progression with less toxicity when compared to patients treated with TACE [44]. Randomized control trials comparing TACE and radioembolization are needed but however are not always possible or technically feasible. At this time, radioembolization has been shown to demonstrate successful tumor downstaging and can help patients who are outside transplant criteria to be downstaged to allow transplantation [45]. In addition, radio-embolization has been shown to be the preferred treatment over TACE in the setting of bulky disease burden as radioembolization results in decreased toxicity and hepatic decompensation [16].

Embolization of Other Tumors

Bland or chemoembolization can be used in the treatment of liver cancers other than HCC including cholangiocarcinoma, angiosarcoma, or metastatic disease from a variety of primary cancers such as colorectal and breast cancer, renal cell mela-noma, or neuroendocrine tumors. The selection criteria are similar to that for patients with HCC, and the goal is to provide symptomatic relief or improvement in survival. In the setting of neuroendocrine tumors, embolization can be extremely beneficial in the treatment of symptoms related to hormone excess. In general, patients with metastatic disease involving the liver are less likely to have advanced cirrhosis as compared to those patients with HCC; therefore there are relatively few contraindications to treatment. The presence of extensive hepatic disease, involving >50–75% of the hepatic parenchyma with the presence of progressive extrahepatic disease is a contraindication to treatment.

Colorectal cancer is the third most common cancer accounting for 10% of total cancer deaths in the United States. These deaths are attributed to metastatic disease rather than the primary tumor. Select patients may be eligible to undergo hepatic resection if they have isolated metastatic disease; however, these patients often develop new tumors due to the micrometastatic and multifocal nature of this illness. Ablative strategies have been used with success in select populations, but high local recurrence rates are seen, particularly in those tumors that are larger than 3.0 cm in diameter [28]. There are also promising data showing benefits of intra-arterial thera-pies, including TACE and radioembolization, in metastatic colorectal cancer to the liver.

Hepatic Trauma

Overview

A multidisciplinary team approach to the trauma patient helps to ensure the most suitable diagnostic evaluation and management decisions are made. The interven-tional radiologist can play a valuable role in that team equipped with the ability to discuss relevant imaging findings and discuss the potential role for endovascular treatment strategies. Provided the patient is reasonably hemodynamically stable,

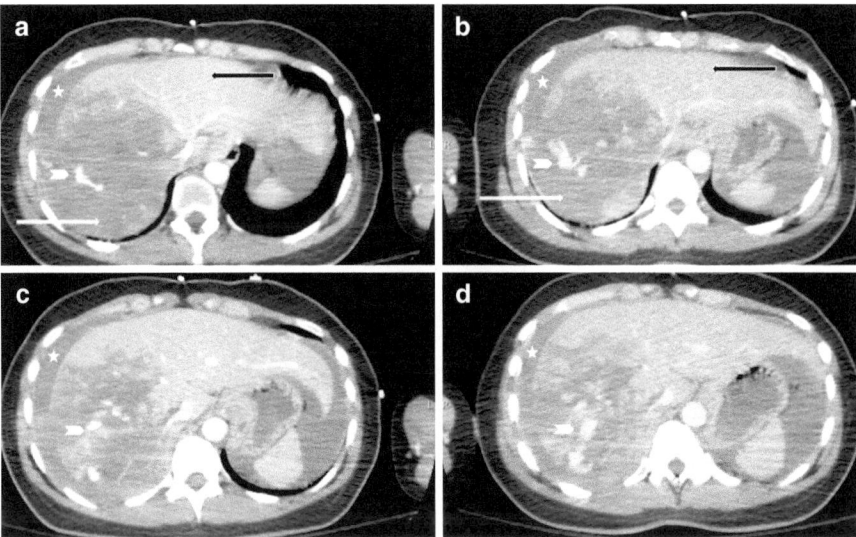

Fig. 8.11 Axial contrast-enhanced CT of the abdomen in the setting of trauma demonstrating a patient with a high-grade liver laceration. (**a**) Axial contrast-enhanced image of the abdomen in the arterial phase denotes the presence of active arterial extravasation, denoted by the arrowhead. In addition, there is a relative lack of perfusion to the right lobe of the liver, as denoted by the white arrow, compared to the left lobe, denoted by the black arrow. A peri-hepatic hematoma is seen denoted by the star symbol. (**b**) Axial CT of the abdomen in the delayed venous phase at the same level as image (**a**), shows the active contrast extravasation denoted by the arrowhead. (**c**) Axial contrast-enhanced CT of the abdomen in the arterial phase slightly more inferior to image (**a**) shows an additional area of active arterial extravasation, denoted by the arrowhead. (**d**) Axial CT of the abdomen in the delayed venous phase at the same level as image (**c**), demonstrates continued contrast extravasation

noninvasive imaging with computed tomography (CT) provides high diagnostic value. Technical advances, reduced scan time, and increased availability of multidetector CT scanners have helped to increase the role of noninvasive imaging in the setting of trauma. CT's provide detailed anatomic information that can be invaluable in the assessment of trauma patients and can be used to direct optimal management [46]. In the setting of suspected abdominal trauma, initial diagnostic imaging should be with a contrast-enhanced CT. Typical protocols include delayed phase imaging which helps differentiate active bleeding from contained vascular injuries (see Figs. 8.11 and 8.12). Although abdominal ultrasound can be performed quickly, there is a high rate of misdiagnosis and therefore should be reserved for hemodynamically unstable patients who cannot receive a CT [47].

There are many types of hepatic trauma including blunt trauma, crush injuries, deceleration injuries, and iatrogenic vascular injuries related to surgeries or procedures such as biopsies. The accurate identification of active arterial bleeding or ischemic end-organ injury is paramount.

Fig. 8.12 Coronal contrast-enhanced CT of the abdomen in the setting of trauma demonstrating a patient with a high-grade liver laceration. A, Coronal contrast-enhanced CT of the abdomen demonstrates the active arterial extravasation, denoted by the arrowhead, the large area of decreased hepatic perfusion seen as parenchymal hypo-density denoted by the thick white arrow, and the presence of the large peri-hepatic hematoma, denoted by the star symbol

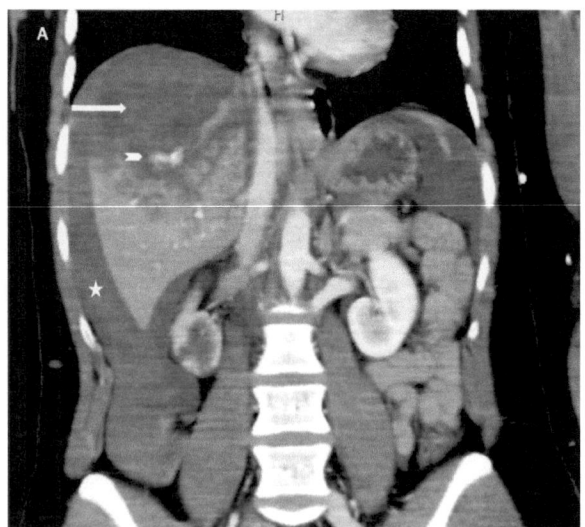

Patient Selection

The approach to treatment of the trauma patient has been defined by the recommendations from the advanced trauma life support (ATLS), which suggests a comprehensive assessment with rapid intervention to achieve hemodynamic stability. The liver is the most commonly injury solid organ occurring in 15–20% of abdominal injuries. Hepatic injury occurs in the setting of both blunt and penetrating trauma and carries an overall mortality of 10% [48]. The American Association for the Surgery of Trauma has detailed a liver injury scale that is useful for categorizing trauma and assists with facilitating patient management and ensuring effective team communication. In general, level I and II are considered minor hepatic trauma and are commonly managed conservatively with supportive measures. In the hemodynamically unstable patient, management should proceed with timely exploratory laparotomy. With the advances in catheter-directed interventional radiology therapies, the management of intermediate hepatic trauma has evolved.

Indications for urgent catheter-based therapies include the finding of active arterial extravasation or clinical suspicion for continued active hemorrhage after exploratory laparotomy or other intervention. Catheter-based interventions can be performed for pseudoaneurysms larger than 5 mm or the finding of AV fistulas in the non-emergent setting when the patient is stable and other traumatic injuries have been addressed.

If the decision for catheter-based intervention has been decided, the patient should undergo the primary and secondary trauma surveys with initial resuscitation prior to arrival to the angiography suite. ATLS guidelines recommend starting resuscitation in adults with volume replacement using two-liter bolus of Ringer's lactate. Throughout the procedure, close monitoring of patient's vital signs with continued adequate resuscitation is required. If after the initial bolus, hemodynamic stability is not yet achieved, further resuscitation efforts should continue with two units of packed red blood cell infusion.

Technique

Prior to performing a catheter-based intervention, a careful review of available imaging should be performed in order to localize the sites of hepatic injury, identify the parent vessel, and investigate for potential collateral vasculature to the area of injury. In addition, the operator must have a thorough knowledge of hepatic arterial anatomy and common variants. The right hepatic artery can commonly arise from the SMA, termed a replaced hepatic artery, and the left hepatic artery can arise from the left gastric artery. Evaluation of the origin of the cystic artery should be performed, as care should be taken to avoid inadvertent embolization.

Angiography is typically performed from transfemoral arterial access with the placement of a 5 French vascular sheath. A thorough diagnostic angiographic evaluation of the patient with hepatic trauma should be performed which includes selective angiograms of the celiac, hepatic, and superior mesenteric arteries. A 4 or 5 French catheter such as a Cobra, Sos, or Simmons catheter can be used to cannulate the visceral vessels. Typical injection parameters for the visceral vessels include the administration of 20–30 mL of contrast at a rate of 5 mL/s. The digital subtraction angiography (DSA) should be carried out for the duration of the arterial, parenchymal, and venous phase to avoid missing a finding of contrast extravasation (see Fig. 8.13). The operator must be well versed in normal hepatic and variant hepatic arterial anatomy. Due to the presence of numerous hepatic collaterals, multiple super-selective angiograms should be performed to reduce the rate of false negative angiograms.

Catheter angiography confirms the suspected diagnosis and source of arterial bleeding with a sensitivity and specificity of 98.3% and 98.5% [49]. False negative angiograms are most commonly secondary to vasospasm, spontaneous thrombus formation, venous bleeding, or artifact obscuring the finding. Angiographic findings of vascular or organ injuries include arterial cutoff, vessel irregularity, intimal flaps or dissection, thrombosis, stagnant pooling of contrast material, diffuse vasoconstriction, pseudoaneurysm, arteriovenous fistula formation, and the presence of a relative avascular intraparenchymal zone.

The catheter-based treatment of a visceral injury commonly involves the embolization of the bleeding source; however occasionally covered stents may be used. Typical embolic agents include particulates such as polyvinyl alcohol (e.g., Bead Block; Biocompatible International, Farnham, UK) and other sphericals (e.g., Embospheres, BioSphere Medical, Inc., Rockland MA; Embozene microspheres; CeloNova BioSciences, Inc., Newnan, GA), absorbable gelatin sponge (Gelfoam;

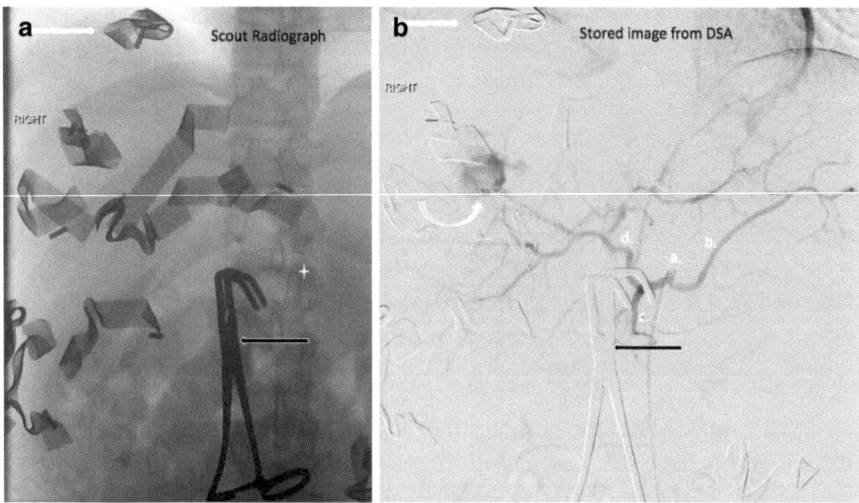

Fig. 8.13 Intra-procedural DSA images of the abdomen in the setting of trauma demonstrating a patient with a high-grade liver laceration. (**a**) Scout radiograph of the abdomen shows the presence of numerous retained surgical sponges, one of which is denoted by the thick white arrow. These surgical sponges have been placed during exploratory laparotomy to pack the abdomen to help control bleeding through a tamponade effect. The large clamp, denoted by the black arrow, is a part of the surgical "Pringle maneuver," whereby the surgeon places an atraumatic hemostat across the hepatoduodenal ligament to interrupt the blood through the hepatic artery and portal vein to attempt to gain control of bleeding. The small white star denotes the site of the angiographic catheter. (**b**) Celiac angiogram performed via the 5Fr catheter. The surgical hemostat has been opened, denoted by the black arrow, allowing blood to flow through the hepatic artery. The celiac axis is denoted by the letter (*a*), the splenic artery denoted by the letter (*b*), the gastroduodenal artery is denoted by the letter (*c*), and the proper hepatic artery is denoted by the letter (*d*). The large area of contrast extravasation is appreciated in the right upper quadrant of the liver denoted by the curved white arrow

Pfizer, Inc., New York, NY), plug occluders, and embolization coils (see Fig. 8.14). The choice of embolic agent is based on anatomic considerations, clinical presentation, and degree of occlusion desired [50]. If multiple vessels are injured, a proximal embolization with Gelfoam may be preferred, particularly in the setting of an unstable patient.

The frequency of posttraumatic hepatic pseudoaneurysm is estimated to be 2–3% and most frequently occurs in patients that sustain a grade 4 hepatic injury. Smaller pseudoaneurysms tend to thrombose without intervention however those larger than 1 cm in size or those that demonstrate rapid enlargement put the patient at increased for a repeat bleed and therefore should be addressed. In many scenarios, interventional radiology can provide a treatment option through the use of selective angiographic coil embolization. Commonly proximal and distal coil embolization, termed "the sandwich technique," is required, as packing of the pseudoaneurysm with coils is not desired due to risk of rupture. Pseudoaneurysms located at the periphery of the liver may not be amenable to intravascular coil embolization but however if large enough may potentially be treated through percutaneous ultrasound-guided transhepatic needle placement with image-guided injection of thrombin. The success rate for treatment of hepatic pseudoaneurysms is around 90%.

Fig. 8.14 Intra-procedural DSA image of the abdomen post Gelfoam embolization of the same patient seen in Fig. 8.13. Stored image from a DSA post-Gelfoam embolization of the proper hepatic artery. The 5Fr parent catheter is in the celiac artery denoted by the letter (*a*), and there is a micro-catheter in the proper hepatic artery denoted by the letter (*b*). Note the surgical hemostat across the hepatoduodenal ligament remains open as denoted by the black arrow. The contrast injection demonstrates no flow into the hepatic arteries post-Gelfoam embolization denoted by the curved white arrow, consistent with angiographic hemostasis

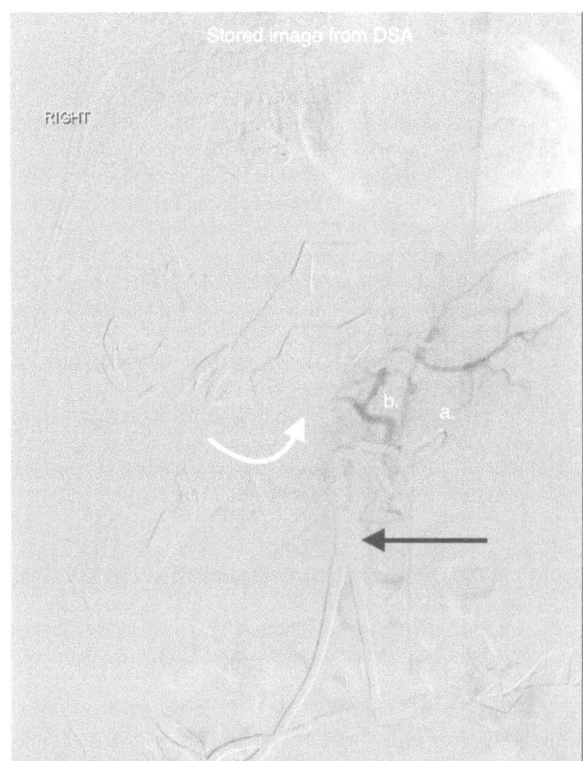

Outcomes

The management of patient's following successful hepatic arterial embolization is largely determined by the extent of the patient's injuries at presentation. In general, the embolization of hepatic arteries is well-tolerated particularly if the patient has a patent portal vein due to the dual blood supply of the liver. The complications of embolotherapy in the setting of hepatic trauma include rebleeding, hepatic infarction, abscess formation, biliary injury, and gallbladder necrosis. As with all arterial interventions, the patient should be monitored after treatment for signs of arterial access-related complications. In the setting of femoral artery access, the patient should remain flat for at least 6 h with pulse checks and site checks performed every 15 min for 1 h, followed by every 30 min for 2 h and then hourly for 2 h. The patient's vital signs should be monitored for evidence of rebleeding. A follow-up CT scan should be performed within 3 weeks to evaluate for pseudoaneurysm.

Catheter-based therapies are an attractive emergency management option in the setting of trauma as they provide a minimally invasive approach and a potentially more directed treatment strategy as compared to an open surgical intervention. The ability to rapidly employ effective treatment strategies through the use of embolotherapy can even be applied to the unstable patient in the proper setting. The benefits of such intervention are it has the ability to quickly control hemorrhage and restore perfusion and thus may result in organ preservation [50].

References

1. Centers for Disease Control and Prevention. National vital statistics reports 1999–2013: chronic liver disease and cirrhosis. 2017. https://urldefense.proofpoint.com/v2/url?u=http-3A__www.cdc.gov_nchs_fastats_liver-2Ddisease.htm&d=DwMFaQ&c=vh6FgFnduejN hPPD0fl_yRaSfZy8CWbWnIf4XJhSqx8&r=43fkppBaj-NTFf-VE6tbGdRVXVBNSGwt-GUrHy3XwlhQ&m=N-jlMHEPo8n2uhLtFVE2i3EKreidel980WqmFXjtfMo&s=v6ZcuSOX Z5zNv_zUVOoBTjrhKDOn0FU5z_Raye12DNw&e=" www.cdc.gov/nchs/fastats/liver-disease.htm. Accessed 5 Sept 2018.
2. Younossi ZM, Stepanova M, Afendy M, et al. Changes in the prevalence of the most common causes of chronic liver diseases in the United States from 1988 to 2008. Clin Gastroenterol Hepatol. 2001;9:5224.
3. Bruix J, Sherman M. Managemetn of hepatocellular carcinoma: an update. Hepatology. 2011;53(3):1020–2.
4. Crocetti L, Bargellini I, Cioni R. Loco-regional treatment of HCC: current status. Clin Radiol. 2017;72:626–35.
5. Forner A, Reig ME, de Lope CR, et al. Current strategy for staging and treatment: the BCLC update and future prospects. Semin Liver Dis. 2010;30(01):61–74.
6. Ozakyol A. Global epidemiology of hepatocellular carcinoma. J Gastrointest Cancer. 2017;48(3):238–40.
7. Kojiro M, Roskams T. Early hepatocellular carcinoma and dysplastic nodules. Semin Liver Dis. 2005;25:133–42.
8. Mitchell DG, Bruix J, Sherman M, et al. LI-RADS: summary, discussion, consensus of the LI-RADS Management Working Group and future directions. Hepatology. 2015;61(3): 1056–65.
9. McEvoy S, McCarthy C, Lavelle L, et al. Hepatocellular carcinoma: illustrated guide to systematic radiologic diagnosis and staging according to guidelines of the American Association for the Study of Liver Disease. Radiographics. 2013;33(6):1653–68.
10. Mitchell DG, Bruix J, Sherman M, Sirlin CB. Liver imaging reporting and data system: summary, discussion and consensus of the LI-RADS Management working group and future. Hepatology. 2015;61(3):1056–65.
11. Freeman RB, Wiesner RH, Harper A, et al. The new liver allocation system: moving toward evidence-based transplantation policy. Liver Transpl. 2002;8(9):851–8.
12. Levy I, Greig PD, Gallinger S, et al. Resection of hepatocellular carcinoma without preoperative tumor biopsy. Ann Surg. 2001;234:206–9.
13. Corcetti L, Bargellini I, Cioni R. Loco-regional treatment of HCC: current status. Clin Radiol. 2017;72:636–5.
14. Bruix J, Reig M, Sherman M. Evidence-based diagnosis, staging and treatment of patients with hepatocellular carcinoma. Gastroenterology. 2016;150(4):835–53.
15. Kokudo N, Hasegawa K, Akahane M, et al. Evidence-based clinical practice guidelines for hepatocellular carcinoma: *The Japan Society of Hepatology*. Hepatol Res. 2015;45(2):123–7.
16. Bolondi L, Burroughs A, Dufour JF, et al. Heterogeneity of patients with intermediate (BCLC B) hepatocellular carcinoma: proposal for sub-classification to facilitate treatment decisions. Semin Liver Dis. 2012;32(4):348–59.
17. Raoul J, Sangro B, Forner A, Mazzaferro V, Piscagelia F, Bolondi L, Lencioni R. Evolving strategies for the managmenet of intermediate-stage hepatocellular carcinoma: available evidence and expert opinion on the use of transarterial chemoembolization. Cancer Treat Rev. 2011;37(3):212–20.
18. Llovet J, Bruix J. Systematic review of randomized trials for unresectable hepatoceullular carcinoma: chemoembolization improves survival. Hepatology. 2003;37(2):429–42.
19. Llovet JM, Fuster J, Bruix J. Intention-to-treat analysis of surgical treatment for early hepatocellular carcinoma: resection versus transplantation. Hepatology. 1999;30:1434–40.
20. Shiina S, Tagawa K, Niwa Y, et al. Percutaneous ethanol injection therapy for hepatocellular carcinoma: results in 146 patients. AJR. 1993;160:1023–8.

21. Lin SM, Lin CJ, Lin CC, et al. Randomized control trial comparing percutaneous radiofrequency thermal ablation, percutaneous ethanol injection and percutaneous acetic acid injection to treat HCC of 3cm or less. Gut. 2005;54(8):1151–6.
22. Yamamoto J, Okada S, Shimada K, et al. Treatment strategy for small hepatocellular carcinoma: comparison of long-term results after percutaneous ethanol injection therapy and surgical resection. Hepatology. 2001;34:707–13.
23. Ahmed M, Brace C, Lee F, Goldberg S. Principles of and advances in percutaneous ablation. Radiology. 2011;258(2):351–69.
24. Mazur P. Freezing of living cells: mechanisms and implications. Am J Physiol. 1984;143:125–42.
25. Sanghvi NT, Hawes RH. High-intensity focused ultrasound. Gastrointestinal Endos Clin North Am. 1994;4(2):383–95.
26. McGahan JP, Dodd GD. Radiofrequency ablation of the liver: current status. AJR Am J Roentgenol. 2001;176:3–16.
27. Wood BK, Ramkaransingh JR, Fojo T, Walther MM, Libutti SK. Percutaneous tumor ablation with radiofrequency. Cancer. 2002;94:443–51.
28. Simon C, Dupuy D, Mayo-Smith W. Microwave ablation: principles and applications. Radiographics. 2005;25(1):S69–83.
29. Skinner M, Iizuka M, Kolios M, Sherar M. A theoretical comparison of energy sources—microwave, ultrasound and laser—for interstitial thermal therapy. Phys Med Biol. 1998;43:3535–47.
30. Edd J, Horowitz L, Davalos R, et al. In vivo results of new focal tissue ablation technique: irreversible electroporation. IEEE Trans Biomed Eng. 2006;53:1409–15.
31. Lo C, Ngan H, Tso W, et al. Randomized controlled trial of transarterial lipiodol chemoembolization for unresectable hepatocellular carcinoma. Hepatology. 2002;35:1164–71.
32. Huang K, Zhou Q, Wang R, et al. Doxorubicin-eluting beads versus conventional transarterial chemoembolization for the treatment of hepatocellular carcinoma. J Gastroenterol Hepatol. 2014;29:920–5.
33. Llovet JM, Real MI, Montana X, et al. Arterial embolization or chemoembolization versus symptomatic treatment in patients with unresectable hepatocellular carcinoma: a randomized controlled trial. Lancet. 2002;359:1734–9.
34. Kawai S, Okamura J, Ogawa M, et al. Prospective and randomized clinical trial for the treatment of hepatocellular carcinoma – a comparison of lipiodol transcatheter arterial embolization with and without adriamycin. Cancer Chemother Pharmacol. 1992;21:1–6.
35. Chang JM, Tzeng WS, Pan HB, et al. Transcatheter arterial embolization with or without cisplatin treatment of hepatocellular carcinoma. A randomized controlled study. Cancer. 1994;74:2449–53.
36. Graziadei IW, Sandmueller H. Chemoembolization followed by liver transplantation for hepatocellular carcinoma impedes tumor progression while on the waiting list and leads to excellent outcome. Liver Transpl. 2003;9:557–63.
37. Llovet JM, Bruix J. A systematic review of randomized control trials for unresectable hepatocellular carcinoma chemoembolization improves survival. Hepatology. 2003;37:429–42.
38. Dawson LA. Hepatic arterial yttrium-90 microspheres: another treatment option for hepatocellular carcinoma. J Vasc Interv Radiol. 2005;16(2):161–4.
39. Popperl G, Helmberger T, Munzing W, et al. Selective internal radiation therapy with SIR-spheres in patients with nonresectable liver tumors. Cancer Biother Radiopharm. 2005;2:200–8.
40. Campbell AM, Bailey IH, Burton MA. Analysis of the distribution of intra-arterial microspheres in human liver following hepatic yttrium-90 microsphere therapy. Phys Med Biol. 2000;4:1023–33.
41. Carretero C, Munoz-Navas M, Betes M, et al. Gastroduodenal injury after radioembolization of hepatic tumors. Am J Gastroenterol. 2007;6:1216–20.
42. Liapi E, Geschwind J-FH. Radioembolization for hepatocellular carcinoma (chapter 65). In: Mauro MA, et al., editors. Image-guided interventions. 2nd ed. Philadelphia: Elsevier; 2014. p. 441–7.
43. Hilgard P, Hamami M, Fouly AE, et al. Radioembolization with ytrrium-90 glass microspheres in hepatocellular carcinoma: European experience on safety and long-term survival. Hepatology. 2010;52(5):1741–9.

44. Salem R, Lewandowski RJ, Mulcahy MF, et al. Radioembolization for hepatocellular carcinoma using yttrium-90 microspheres. A comprehensive report of long-term outcomes. Gastroenterology. 2009;138(1):52–64.
45. Lewandowski RJ, Kulik LM, Riaz A, et al. A comparative analysis of transarterial downstaging for hepatocellular carcinoma: chemoembolization versus radioembolization. Am J Transplant. 2009;9(8):1920–8.
46. Huber-Wagner S, Lefering R, Quick L, et al. Effect of whole-body CT during trauma resuscitation on survival: a retrospective multicenter study. Lancet. 2009;373:1455–61.
47. Yu W-Y, Li Q-J, Gong J-P. Treatment strategy for hepatic trauma. Chin J Traumatol. 2016;19:168–71.
48. Steichen FM. Hepatic trauma in adults. Surg Clin North Am. 1975;55:387–407.
49. Rose SC, Moore EE. Emergency trauma angiography: accuracy, safety and pitfalls. Am J Roentgenol. 1987;148:1243–6.
50. Salazar G, Walker TG. Evaluation and management of acute vascular trauma. Tech Vasc Interv Radiol. 2009;12:102–16.

Chapter 9
Radiologic Diagnosis and Intervention for Gastrointestinal Bleeding

John A. Cieslak, Elena G. Violari, and Charan K. Singh

Introduction

Acute gastrointestinal bleeding (GIB) occurs with an annual incidence of approximately 40–150 cases per 10,000 persons for upper GIB and 20–27 cases per 100,000 persons for lower GIB [1–3]. Gastrointestinal bleeding can be classified into upper or lower gastrointestinal bleeding depending on if the source is proximal or distal to the ligament of Treitz, respectively. The mortality rate for both upper and lower GIB is estimated to be around 4–10% [1–3]. There are multiple etiologies for GIB, which can be categorized generally into infectious, vascular anomalies, inflammatory disease, trauma, and malignancy (Table 9.1) [4–10].

Diagnostic and treatment approach of GIB depends on its location, severity, and etiology [3]. The first line for diagnosis and treatment when GIB is suspected is usually a gastroenterology consult for esophagoduodenoscopy (EGD) or colonoscopy. If a bleeding source is visualized, endoscopic therapy options include epinephrine injection and coaptive coagulation, hemo-clip placement, argon plasma coagulation, sclerotherapy, and band ligation, to name a few [11]. The role of radiology becomes especially important in patients whose GIB remains resistant to medical and endoscopic treatment [3]. Diagnostic imaging studies can be used to effectively localize the source of bleeding. Tests such as CT angiography, ^{99m}Tc-labeled red blood cell

J. A. Cieslak (✉)
Northwestern University Feinberg School of Medicine, Chicago, IL, USA
e-mail: john.cieslak@northwestern.edu

E. G. Violari
Department of Radiology, University of Connecticut Health Center, Farmington, CT, USA
e-mail: violari@uchc.edu

C. K. Singh
Department of Interventional Radiology, University of Connecticut Health Center, Farmington, CT, USA

© Springer International Publishing Switzerland 2018
C. K. Singh (ed.), *Gastrointestinal Interventional Radiology*, Clinical Gastroenterology, https://doi.org/10.1007/978-3-319-91316-2_9

Table 9.1 Common etiologies of upper and lower GI bleeding

Upper GI bleeds	Lower GI bleeds
Esophagitis	Diverticular disease
Gastritis	Hemorrhoids
Peptic ulcer disease	Colitis: inflammatory, infectious, ischemic, radiation
Mallory-Weiss tear	Angiodysplasia
Esophageal varices	Rectal varices
Gastric varices	Polyps/post-polypectomy
Pill ulcer	Intussusception
Foreign bodies	Meckel's diverticulum
Neoplasm	Neoplasm
Coagulopathy	Coagulopathy
Traumatic	Traumatic

scintigraphy (tagged RBC scan), and digital subtraction angiography (DSA) are all options for the detection of GI bleeding, but their sensitivity is largely dependent on the rate of hemorrhage, with DSA only sensitive to rapid bleeding and tagged RBC scans most sensitive for slow bleeds. Once a source of bleeding is identified, endovascular therapeutic interventions such as transcatheter arterial embolization (TAE) can be performed in the interventional radiology suite to achieve hemostasis.

Despite the etiology, initial evaluation of patients with GIB should always begin with a history and physical examination. Focused abdominal exam and digital rectal exam should be performed in any patient with GI bleeding. Tachycardia, orthostatic hypotension, and chronic anemia are all potential signs of GI bleeding [12]. Risk factors for bleeding include anticoagulation (warfarin, NSAIDs, aspirin, corticosteroids), congenital coagulopathy, previous history of GIB, history of abdominal surgery, recent colonoscopy with polypectomy, previous abdominal or pelvic radiation, abdominal aortic aneurysm, history of alcoholism, and chronic renal or liver disease. Family or personal history of colon cancer or inflammatory bowel disease should also be noted.

In hemodynamically unstable patients, two large-bore IVs should be placed, and IV fluid resuscitation and possibly blood products should be administered rapidly to replete intravascular volume and stabilize vital signs [3]. In some patients, correction of coagulopathy may also be needed [13]. Often, diagnostic workup should be occurring simultaneously during resuscitation, to minimize morbidity and mortality associated with GIB [13–15].

Upper Gastrointestinal Bleeding

The incidence of acute upper gastrointestinal bleeding is approximately 40–150 cases per 100,000 persons per year, is twice as common in men compared to women, and increases in prevalence with age [1–3, 16]. Seventy-six percent of all gastrointestinal bleeding events are classified as upper GIB, and the mortality rate is approximately 5%. Classically, patients with upper GIB present with hematemesis or

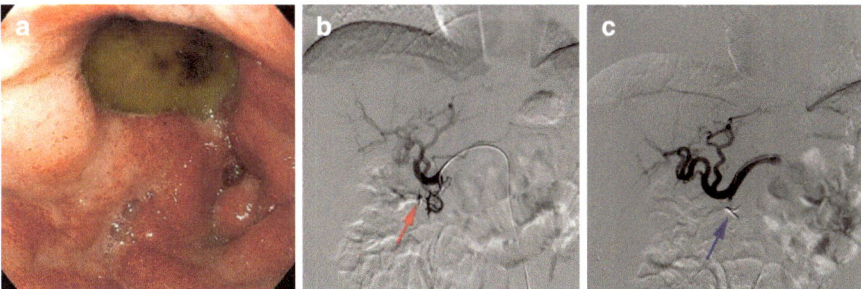

Fig. 9.1 Bleeding and intervention in a patient with peptic ulcer disease. (**a**) Endoscopic view of a duodenal ulcer, suspected source of the patient's upper GI bleed, though not actively bleeding at the time this picture was taken. (**b**) Digital subtraction gastroduodenal artery (GDA) angiography showing opacification of the proximal GDA with active extravasation at the site of ulceration (red arrow). (**c**) Digital subtraction GDA angiography images demonstrating cessation of bleeding (absence of blush) after glue embolization of the GDA, which is no longer opacified (blue arrow)

melena, though 15% of patients still present with hematochezia, indicating that the bleeding is brisk [14, 16, 17]. Gastric lavage with NG tube insertion can be performed to investigate whether upper GIB is prepyloric, but a negative result does not completely exclude it. Additionally, upper GIB distal to the pylorus will not be detected with gastric lavage. Studies estimate that approximately 25–60% of upper GIB is secondary to peptic ulcer disease (Fig. 9.1a) [16]. This is often associated with nonsteroidal anti-inflammatory (NSAID) drug use and/or *Helicobacter pylori* infection [15, 18]. If the patient has known peptic ulcer disease and is having hematemesis, EGD is always performed first to see if a bleeding ulcer can be identified and treated endoscopically. However, if there is failure in treating the bleeding gastric ulcer endoscopically, interventional radiology will commonly embolize the gastroduodenal artery (GDA), the most likely artery to be involved in supplying the ulcerated mucosa of the stomach, even in the absence of extravasation on angiography (Fig. 9.1b, c). Due to the rich collateral blood supply to the stomach, it is important to occlude the backend of the GDA in addition to its origin ("closing the back door"), as well as occluding collaterals from the pancreaticoduodenal artery and gastroepiploic arcade, which can cause back bleeding. The second most common cause of upper GIB is bleeding from varices (esophageal and gastric) [19] in the setting of cirrhosis of the liver. Additional etiologies include gastritis, esophagitis, and duodenitis; cancer (esophageal, gastric, and GIST); mechanical (Mallory-Weiss tear and trauma); vascular abnormalities (vascular ectasia, angiodysplasia, and vascular malformations); aorto-duodenal fistula; and iatrogenic causes.

Lower Gastrointestinal Bleeding

Lower GIB occurs less commonly than upper GIB with an incidence of approximately 20 cases per 100,000 persons per year but is also more common in men and older individuals [20]. Lower GIB is estimated to account for 1–2% of hospital emergencies in the United States. Approximately, 80–85% of lower GI bleeds originate distal to the ileocecal valve, with only 0.7–9% originating from the small intestine [21]. The most common presentation of lower GIB is hematochezia. Less commonly, patients may present with melena if the source of bleeding is located in the small bowel or right colon [3]. Diverticulosis is the most common cause of painless hematochezia (40% of cases), with the incidence increasing with ages older than 65. Hemorrhoids are the most common cause of lower GIB in patients younger than 50. Other causes include inflammatory bowel disease, ischemic colitis, neoplasia, polyps, vascular malformations, post-polypectomy, and angiodysplasia [3, 12, 21, 22]. Although more than 80% of lower GIB will stop spontaneously with conservative management, 10–15% of cases eventually require endovascular intervention [23]. Overall mortality has been noted to be 2–4% [21].

Endoscopy

Endoscopy is the first choice for diagnosis and therapy in both upper and lower gastrointestinal bleeding, and therefore consultation with gastroenterology should not be delayed when a patient presents with GIB. In patients with upper GI bleed, EGD is performed; in patients with suspected lower GI bleed, colonoscopy is the procedure of choice. Colonoscopy has been shown to correctly identify the source of lower GIB in more than 75% of patients while also allowing a therapeutic modality [21]. Factors that may predict endoscopic treatment failure include patients that present with shock, hemoglobin less than 10, greater than six units of blood transfused, and significant comorbidities [3]. Additionally, lack of bowel preparation may limit the ability of colonoscopy to identify the source of bleeding, or blood may be seen within the colon lumen, but the exact site of bleeding may be difficult to identify [24].

The Role of Diagnostic Imaging Studies in the Diagnosis and Localization of Gastrointestinal Bleeding

When a patient has nondiagnostic endoscopic results or remains refractory to medical and endoscopic treatment, radiologic imaging and endovascular intervention are the next intervention of choice [3]. CT angiography and ^{99m}Tc-labeled red blood cell scintigraphy (tagged RBC scan) are noninvasive options available for the diagnosis and localization of GIB, but it is important to remember that these are diagnostic only and that bleeding will still have to be treated with subsequent endovascular or surgical intervention after localization.

Table 9.2 Comparison of imaging modalities for the detection of gastrointestinal bleeding

	CT angiography	Tagged RBC scan	DS angiography
Sensitivity	85%	95%	60%
Specificity	99%	93%	100%
Rates of bleeding detected	0.3–0.5 mL/min	0.1–0.35 mL/min	0.5–1.0 mL/min
Detection of intermittent bleeding	No	Yes	No
Therapeutic	No	No	Potentially

CT Angiography

CT angiography (CTA) is relatively noninvasive, fast and widely available, and relatively effective at detecting GIB in patients with continuous bleeding [25]. CTA can detect bleeding rates of 0.3–0.5 mL/min (Table 9.2), has a relatively low sensitivity (85–90%) [21], but a specificity of 99% and an accuracy of 97.6% in localizing both upper and lower GI bleeds. CTA exams obtained for GIB are usually three-phase studies, including unenhanced (non-contrast), arterial phase, and portal venous phase images. Slice thickness is normally thin (1 mm) and tube voltage high (120 kV) to improve the sensitivity and contrast of the study, but imaging parameters vary slightly depending on institution. On unenhanced images, focal hyperattenuation within the bowel is indicative of recent hemorrhage and may represent a "sentinel clot" [26]. On arterial phase, extravasation of free contrast (extraluminal contrast) is the hallmark of active bleeding and is used to identify/localize the source. Two cases of lower GI bleeding detected on CTA secondary to stercoral ulceration (Fig. 9.2a) and sigmoid diverticulosis (Fig. 9.3a) are shown. Furthermore, a changing appearance of the focus of extravasated contrast between the arterial and portal venous phase indicates active bleeding [27]. Because CTA detection of GIB depends on the identification of free contrast or a sentinel clot, oral contrast is withheld during this study as it can mask the source of bleeding. Again, while not therapeutic, CTA is useful to identify and localize the source of GIB and can also characterize the patient's vascular anatomy, which can be used for surgical or endovascular planning. However, certain patient factors such as contrast allergy and acute/chronic kidney disease are potential contraindications to CT angiography, which uses more contrast than conventional DSA angiography.

^{99m}Tc-Labeled RBC Nuclear Scintigraphy (Tagged RBC Scan)

In ^{99m}Tc-labeled RBC nuclear scintigraphy, erythrocytes are labeled with technetium-99m, infused into the patient, and then serial scintigraphy is performed to detect focal collections of radiolabeled material within the GI tract (i.e., sites of GI

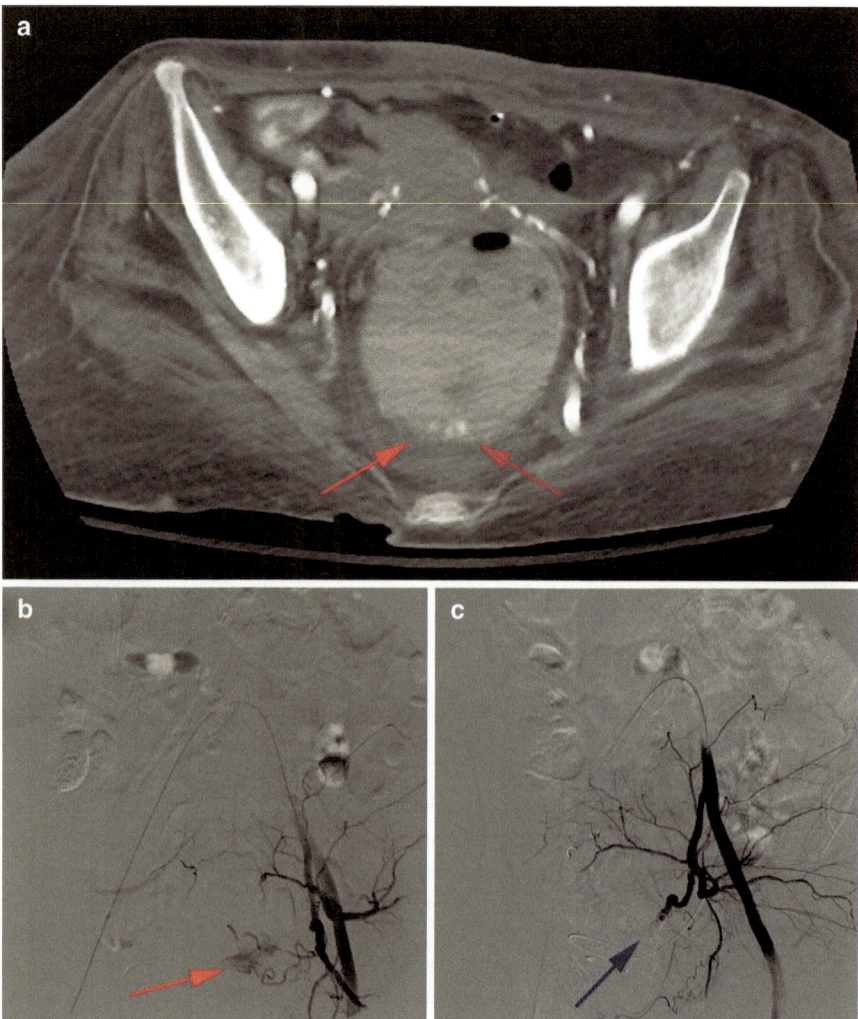

Fig. 9.2 Bleeding and intervention in a chronically constipated patient with stercoral ulcer. (**a**) CTA demonstrating active extravasation of contrast in the dependent portion of the rectum (red arrows), indicative of active lower GI bleeding. (**b**) Digital subtraction angiography images demonstrating active extravasation of contrast (red arrow) from the left middle rectal artery. (**c**) Digital subtraction angiography images demonstrating cessation of bleeding (absence of blush) after coil embolization of the left middle rectal artery (blue arrow)

bleeding). Nuclear scintigraphy is a valuable imaging modality for the detection of slow lower GI bleeding, with bleeding rates as low as 0.1–0.35 mL/min able to be detected (Table 9.2) [28]. The overall sensitivity and specificity of Tc-99m-labeled red blood cell studies are 95% and 93%, respectively [29]. Additionally, nuclear scintigraphy is advantageous in that it allows for continuous monitoring and can

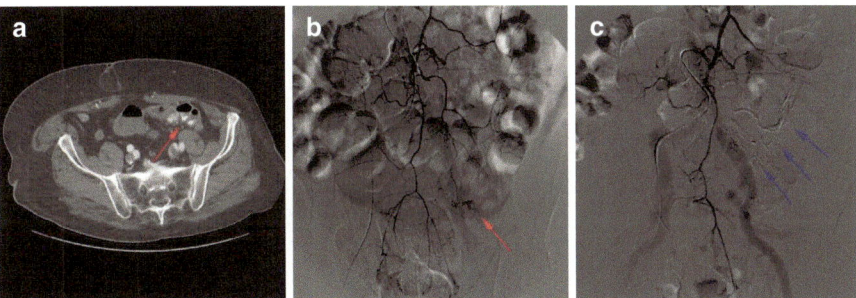

Fig. 9.3 Bleeding and intervention in a patient with diverticulosis. (**a**) CTA demonstrating active extravasation of contrast in the sigmoid colon at a diverticulum (red arrow), indicative of active lower GI bleeding. (**b**) Digital subtraction angiography images demonstrating active extravasation of contrast (red arrow) from the sigmoid branch of the inferior mesenteric artery. (**c**) Digital subtraction angiography images demonstrating cessation of bleeding (absence of blush) after Gelfoam slurry embolization into the IMA (blue arrows)

detect and localize sites of intermittent bleeding which is a common characteristic of lower GIB. The half-life of ^{99m}Tc is long so the scan can be repeated several times in a 24 hour period to evaluate sequential images [21]. Another advantage is that nuclear scintigraphy can help predict which patient will benefit from subsequent angiography. Patients with immediate blush on red blood cell scintigraphy (time to positive (TTP) less than 9 min, Fig. 9.4) are more likely to require urgent angiography, and those with delayed blush (TTP greater than 9 min) have low angiographic yield [3, 30].

Digital Subtraction Angiography

In emergent cases when patients are hemodynamically unstable, or in hospitals where CTA or nuclear scintigraphy is not available, patients with active GI bleeding who fail medical and endoscopic intervention should undergo endovascular angiographic evaluation [3]. Angiography is well suited for the detection of active and fairly brisk lower GI bleeds. Indeed, out of the imaging modalities discussed above, it is the least sensitive and requires bleeding rates of 0.5–1.0 mL/min for positive detection and localization (Table 9.2) [31, 32]. For lower GIB, angiography performed with digital subtraction has an overall sensitivity of 60% and specificity of 100% [3]. Digital subtraction angiography (DSA) is used to better visualize the vasculature by subtracting pre-contrast image from later images and effectively removing soft tissue and bones from the images (Figs. 9.2b and 9.5b); however, this technique is limited by peristalsis or patient breathing [3]. DSA is unique in that it is also potentially therapeutic at the time of diagnosis, allowing for selective embolization of the bleeding vessel. However, certain patient factors such as contrast allergy and acute/chronic kidney disease are potential contraindications to angiography.

Fig. 9.4 ⁹⁹ᵐTc-labeled
RBC nuclear scintigraphy
(tagged RBC scan)
demonstrating uptake and
immediate blush in the
expected region of the
descending colon (red
arrow), indicative of
positive lower GI bleed.
The patient was referred
for urgent mesenteric
angiography

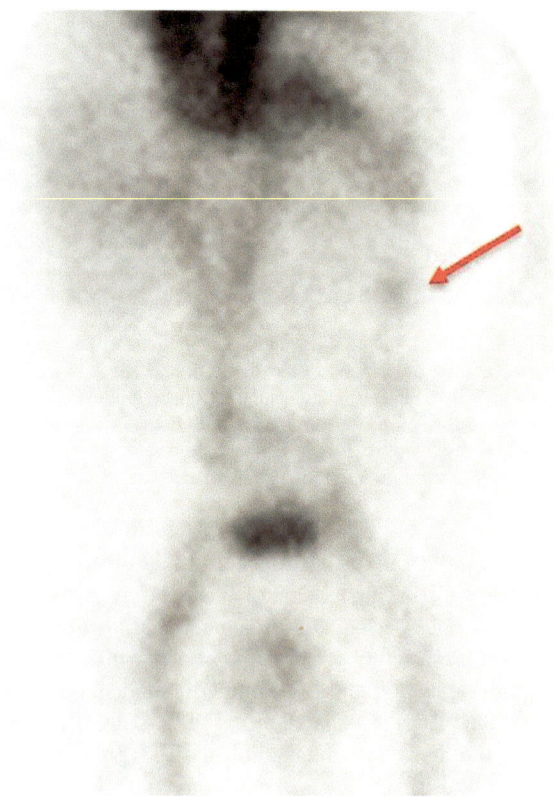

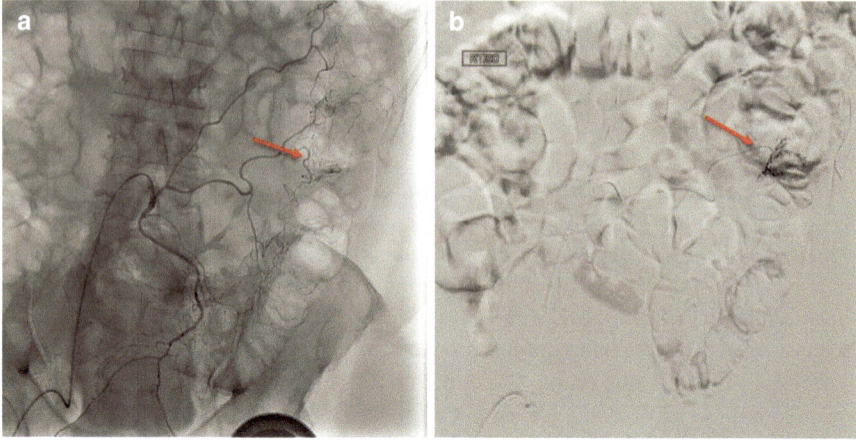

Fig. 9.5 Inferior mesenteric angiography images without (**a**) and with (**b**) digital subtraction demonstrating active extravasation of contrast (red arrows) in a subselective branch along the descending colon, indicating an active lower GI bleed

Access for endovascular angiography is gained via the common femoral artery [33, 34]. The suspected bleeding artery (based on prior imaging studies—if available) is then selectively catheterized and interrogated first. For upper GIB, the celiac, left gastric, and gastroduodenal arteries are studied. If lower GIB is suspected, the branches of the superior mesenteric artery are evaluated first (small bowel and proximal colon are evaluated), and if no source of bleeding is identified, the branches of the inferior mesenteric artery are studied (evaluates colon distal to the splenic flexure). Extravasation of contrast agent (blush) is indicative of active bleeding (Figs. 9.2b, 9.3b, and 9.5a, b) [34]. In Fig. 9.2b, a blush of active contrast extravasation from the middle rectal artery indicates an active and brisk bleed—in this case secondary to stercoral ulcer, as discussed above. In Fig. 9.3b, a blush of active contrast extravasation from the sigmoid branch of the IMA also indicates an active, brisk bleed—in this case secondary to diverticulosis, as discussed above. Positive findings include mucosal blushes with abnormal vessels suggestive of tumor, prolonged contrast spots suggestive of inflammation, and visualization of arteries and veins on the same phase of the study suggestive of an arteriovenous malformation [3]. It is important to keep in mind that active extravasation may not always be seen on angiography, but other findings during the study may suggest the source of bleeding. Examples of this include visualization of varices in unexpected locations or abnormal clusters of vessels within the bowel wall (angiodysplasia). Additionally, intermittent bleeding, venous bleeding, failure to inject the correct artery, or bleeding outside the field of view of the study are additional considerations for a negative study. Repeat examination and subselective catheterization may have to be performed if the patient continues to bleed after a negative angiogram.

Angiographic Interventions in Gastrointestinal Bleeding

As discussed above, endovascular angiography is an effective diagnostic modality for the detection of gastrointestinal bleeding, but it also has the advantage of being a therapeutic tool as well through transcatheter arterial embolization (TAE) and is a safe alternative to surgical intervention in patients who have GIB refractory to medical and endoscopic treatment [3, 35]. Using this technique, hemostasis is achieved by reducing blood flow to the bleeding vessel via injection of particles or other embolic materials (see below), thus decreasing perfusion pressure and facilitating clot formation at the site of bleeding [36, 37].

Transcatheter Arterial Embolization

TAE has been demonstrated to be a safe and effective method for controlling GIB in patients who have failed medical and endoscopic treatment, as well as in patients who are not ideal candidates for endoscopic or surgical interventions. The goal of

TAE is to embolize the bleeding vessels to reduce arterial perfusion pressure and promote clotting. As a consequence of this, one of the major potential complications of TAE is bowel ischemia/infarction. The bowel distal to the ligament of Treitz (lower GIBs) does not have a dual supply; therefore, the risk of bowel infarction is higher [37, 38]. This risk is minimized by super-selecting the most distal branch of the involved artery as possible (vasa recta, Fig. 9.6), as to reduce perfusion pressure while maintaining adequate collateral blood flow to the bowel [36]. Unlike the lower GI blood supply, there is a rich collateral network in the upper bowel (proximal to the ligament of Treitz), so bowel ischemia is less likely. In fact, there is actually a high incidence of rebleeding in upper GIB, due to this collateral supply.

Typically, a 5 French catheter would be used to access the celiac, superior mesenteric artery or inferior mesenteric artery, and a smaller coaxial 3 French microcatheter advanced through it over a 0.018 in guidewire until it is in a super-selective position (Fig. 9.7a, b). Additional potential complications of TAE include vessel perforation, dissection, and vasospasm. Once the microcatheter is in a super-selective position, embolic agents are deployed to induce clotting.

The type of embolic agent used is dependent on experience and preference, the etiology of bleeding, and availability of the agent [3]. Common agents include glue, Gelfoam, coils, PVA particles, and Amplatzer vascular plugs [39–41]. Coils are composed of a metallic component, which acts to physically occlude the vessel, and a fibrotic component that promotes clotting; they come in a variety of shapes and sizes (Fig. 9.8a, b). Figure 9.2c demonstrates successful deployment of coils (blue arrow) within the previously identified bleeding middle rectal artery (secondary to stercoral ulcer), resulting in cessation of the bleed. The advantage of using microcoils is that they can be visualized under direct fluoroscopy and they permit decreased perfusion pressure while preserving collateral flow to prevent infarction.

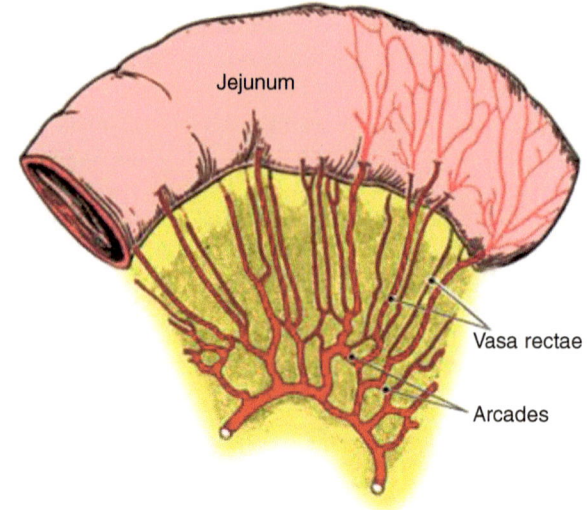

Fig. 9.6 The bowel distal to the ligament of Treitz does not have a dual supply; the vasa recta represent the terminal arterial circulation proximal to the arterioles and should be super-selected for embolization in GI bleeding to reduce perfusion pressure while maintaining adequate collateral blood flow to the bowel, minimizing the chance of bowel ischemia (Image Copyright © 2004–2013 Duke University School of Medicine)

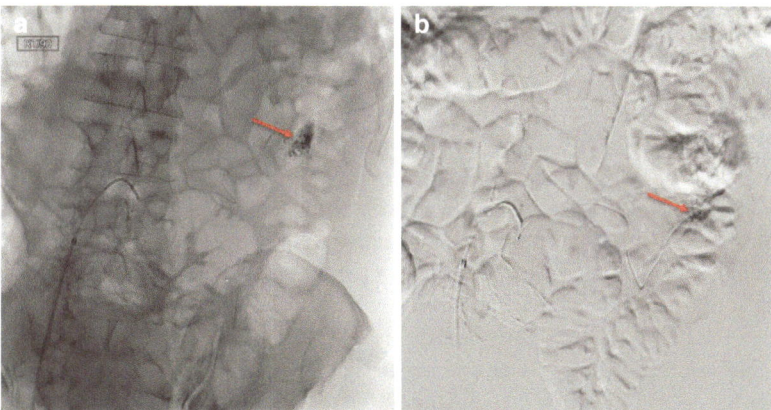

Fig. 9.7 Super-selective catheterization and angiography of the bleeding vessel shown in Fig. 9.5 without (**a**) and with (**b**) digital subtraction, demonstrating active extravasation of contrast (red arrows). 500–700 μm embospheres were utilized to embolize the small super-selective IMA branch

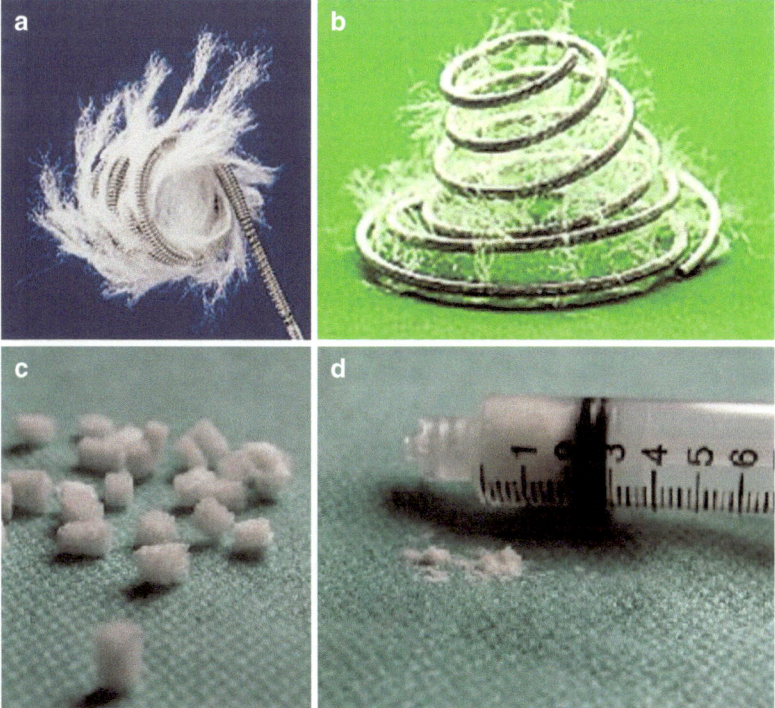

Fig. 9.8 Embolic agents. Metal coils (**a**) and (**b**) cause occlusion as a result of coil-induced thrombosis rather than mechanical occlusion of the lumen by the coil. To increase the thrombogenic effect, Dacron wool tails are attached to coils. The coils are available in many sizes and may be delivered through commonly used angiographic catheters. Gelfoam pledgets (**c**) and slurry (**d**). Gelfoam pledgets are mixed with contrast solution in a syringe forming a slurry, which is then injected slowly under fluoroscopic guidance

Gelfoam is a temporary thrombotic agent comprised of subcutaneous porcine adipose tissue that remains effective for weeks to months before recanalization occurs [3]. Gelfoam is widely available, is cost-effective, and allows future access to embolized vessels after resorption (Fig. 9.8c, d). However, a disadvantage of Gelfoam is that since it is comprised of small particulates, its placement can be unpredictable and has higher risk of bowel ischemia due to unintended distal migration and occlusion at the arteriolar level distal to the level of collateralization (Fig. 9.3c) [34]. Additionally, recanalization times after Gelfoam occlusion are often unpredictable, and therefore it is not recommended as a single embolic agent. Indeed, several studies have shown that recurrent bleeding is more likely to occur when PVA particles, Gelfoam, or coils are used alone [39, 41, 42].

Glues such as N-butyl-2-cyanoacrylate (NBCA) or ethylene-vinyl alcohol copolymer have several advantages including the ability to occlude vessels beyond the most distal site of microcatheter advancement (Fig. 9.1c), permanent vessel closure, the option for using ultra-microcatheters not suitable for microcoil delivery, more efficient obliteration of bleeding pseudoaneurysms with complex anatomy, and lower rebleeding rates than coils or particles [3]. However, they are significantly more expensive and pose a risk for glue reflux, nontarget embolization, bowel infarction, and future bowel stenosis [43]. Clinical success rates of embolization for upper GIB have been cited to range from 44% to 100%, whereas reported success rates for embolization of lower GIB range from 88% to 93% [35, 36, 39, 44].

References

1. Longstreth GF. Epidemiology and outcome of patients hospitalized with acute lower gastrointestinal hemorrhage: a population-based study. Am J Gastroenterol. 1997;92(3):419–24.
2. Manning-Dimmitt LL, Dimmitt SG, Wilson GR. Diagnosis of gastrointestinal bleeding in adults. Am Fam Physician. 2005;71(7):1339–46.
3. Ramaswamy RS, et al. Role of interventional radiology in the management of acute gastrointestinal bleeding. World J Radiol. 2014;6(4):82–92.
4. Boonpongmanee S, et al. The frequency of peptic ulcer as a cause of upper-GI bleeding is exaggerated. Gastrointest Endosc. 2004;59(7):788–94.
5. Cook DJ, et al. Risk factors for gastrointestinal bleeding in critically ill patients. Canadian Critical Care Trials Group. N Engl J Med. 1994;330(6):377–81.
6. Enestvedt BK, Gralnek IM, Mattek N, Lieberman DA, Eisen G. An evaluation of endoscopic indications and findings related to nonvariceal upper-GI hemorrhage in a large multicenter consortium. Gastrointest Endosc. 2008;67(3):422–9.
7. Hreinsson JP, Kalaitzakis E, Gudmundsson S, Bjornsson ES. Upper gastrointestinal bleeding: incidence, etiology and outcomes in a population-based setting. Scand J Gastroenterol. 2013;48(4):439–47.
8. Longstreth GF. Epidemiology of hospitalization for acute upper gastrointestinal hemorrhage: a population-based study. Am J Gastroenterol. 1995;90(2):206–10.
9. van Leerdam ME. Epidemiology of acute upper gastrointestinal bleeding. Best Pract Res Clin Gastroenterol. 2008;22(2):209–24.
10. Zuccaro G. Epidemiology of lower gastrointestinal bleeding. Best Pract Res Clin Gastroenterol. 2008;22(2):225–32.

11. Hui AJ, Sung JJ. Endoscopic treatment of upper gastrointestinal bleeding. Curr Treat Options Gastroenterol. 2005;8(2):153–62.
12. Strate LL, Orav EJ, Syngal S. Early predictors of severity in acute lower intestinal tract bleeding. Arch Intern Med. 2003;163(7):838–43.
13. Ahmed A, Stanley AJ. Acute upper gastrointestinal bleeding in the elderly: aetiology, diagnosis and treatment. Drugs Aging. 2012;29(12):933–40.
14. Barkun A, Bardou M, Marshall JK, Nonvariceal Upper GI Bleeding Consensus Conference Group. Consensus recommendations for managing patients with nonvariceal upper gastrointestinal bleeding. Ann Intern Med. 2003;139(10):843–57.
15. Barnert J, Messmann H. Diagnosis and management of lower gastrointestinal bleeding. Nat Rev Gastroenterol Hepatol. 2009;6(11):637–46.
16. Wilkins T, Khan N, Nabh A, Schade RR. Diagnosis and management of upper gastrointestinal bleeding. Am Fam Physician. 2012;85(5):469–76.
17. Srygley FD, Gerardo CJ, Tran T, Fisher DA. Does this patient have a severe upper gastrointestinal bleed? JAMA. 2012;307(10):1072–9.
18. Kerlin MP, Tokar JL. Acute gastrointestinal bleeding. Ann Intern Med. 2013;159(11):793–4.
19. Lu Y, Loffroy R, Lau JY, Barkun A. Multidisciplinary management strategies for acute nonvariceal upper gastrointestinal bleeding. Br J Surg. 2014;101(1):e34–50.
20. Jang BI. Lower gastrointestinal bleeding: is urgent colonoscopy necessary for all hematochezia? Clin Endosc. 2013;46(5):476–9.
21. Amin SK, Antunes C. Gastrointestinal bleeding, lower. Treasure Island: StatPearls; 2017.
22. Strate LL. Lower GI bleeding: epidemiology and diagnosis. Gastroenterol Clin North Am. 2005;34(4):643–64.
23. Billingham RP. The conundrum of lower gastrointestinal bleeding. Surg Clin North Am. 1997;77(1):241–52.
24. Zuckerman GR, Prakash C, Askin MP, Lewis BS. AGA technical review on the evaluation and management of occult and obscure gastrointestinal bleeding. Gastroenterology. 2000;118(1):201–21.
25. Geffroy Y, et al. Multidetector CT angiography in acute gastrointestinal bleeding: why, when, and how. Radiographics. 2011;31(3):E35–46.
26. Orwig D, Federle MP. Localized clotted blood as evidence of visceral trauma on CT: the sentinel clot sign. AJR Am J Roentgenol. 1989;153(4):747–9.
27. Artigas JM, et al. Multidetector CT angiography for acute gastrointestinal bleeding: technique and findings. Radiographics. 2013;33(5):1453–70.
28. Ford PV, et al. Procedure guideline for gastrointestinal bleeding and Meckel's diverticulum scintigraphy. Society of Nuclear Medicine. J Nucl Med. 1999;40(7):1226–32.
29. Bunker SR, et al. Scintigraphy of gastrointestinal hemorrhage: superiority of 99mTc red blood cells over 99mTc sulfur colloid. AJR Am J Roentgenol. 1984;143(3):543–8.
30. Ng DA, et al. Predictive value of technetium Tc 99m-labeled red blood cell scintigraphy for positive angiogram in massive lower gastrointestinal hemorrhage. Dis Colon Rectum. 1997;40(4):471–7.
31. Winzelberg GG, et al. Radionuclide localization of lower gastrointestinal hemorrhage. Radiology. 1981;139(2):465–9.
32. Zuckerman GR, Prakash C. Acute lower intestinal bleeding. Part II: etiology, therapy, and outcomes. Gastrointest Endosc. 1999;49(2):228–38.
33. Navuluri R, Patel J, Kang L. Role of interventional radiology in the emergent management of acute upper gastrointestinal bleeding. Semin Interv Radiol. 2012;29(3):169–77.
34. Walker TG, Salazar GM, Waltman AC. Angiographic evaluation and management of acute gastrointestinal hemorrhage. World J Gastroenterol. 2012;18(11):1191–201.
35. Yap FY, et al. Transcatheter embolotherapy for gastrointestinal bleeding: a single center review of safety, efficacy, and clinical outcomes. Dig Dis Sci. 2013;58(7):1976–84.
36. Evangelista PT, Hallisey MJ. Transcatheter embolization for acute lower gastrointestinal hemorrhage. J Vasc Interv Radiol. 2000;11(5):601–6.

37. Funaki B. On-call treatment of acute gastrointestinal hemorrhage. Semin Interv Radiol. 2006;23(3):215–22.
38. Funaki B, et al. Superselective microcoil embolization of colonic hemorrhage. AJR Am J Roentgenol. 2001;177(4):829–36.
39. Aina R, et al. Arterial embolotherapy for upper gastrointestinal hemorrhage: outcome assessment. J Vasc Interv Radiol. 2001;12(2):195–200.
40. Loffroy R, et al. Arterial embolotherapy for endoscopically unmanageable acute gastroduodenal hemorrhage: predictors of early rebleeding. Clin Gastroenterol Hepatol. 2009;7(5):515–23.
41. Loffroy R, et al. Short- and long-term results of transcatheter embolization for massive arterial hemorrhage from gastroduodenal ulcers not controlled by endoscopic hemostasis. Can J Gastroenterol. 2009;23(2):115–20.
42. Loffroy RF, Abualsaud BA, Lin MD, Rao PP. Recent advances in endovascular techniques for management of acute nonvariceal upper gastrointestinal bleeding. World J Gastrointest Surg. 2011;3(7):89–100.
43. Lang EK. Transcatheter embolization in management of hemorrhage from duodenal ulcer: long-term results and complications. Radiology. 1992;182(3):703–7.
44. Mirsadraee S, Tirukonda P, Nicholson A, Everett SM, McPherson SJ. Embolization for non-variceal upper gastrointestinal tract haemorrhage: a systematic review. Clin Radiol. 2011;66(6):500–9.

Index